EFFECTIVE BALANCE EXERCISES FOR SENIORS

7 QUICK AND EASY FITNESS ROUTINES TO HELP IMPROVE BALANCE AND FLEXIBILITY

MIKE BRADY

CONTENTS

INTRODUCTION

I don't know about you, but I have reached an age when I can allow myself to indulge in various ways. When I was young, I scoffed at growing old as it was so far in the future that I didn't have to worry about it. But boy, oh boy, those years just flew in many ways. When I was young, I scoffed at growing old as it was so far in the future that I didn't have to worry about it. But boy, oh boy, those years just flew by, and now I sit with, and now I sit with the legacy of my youth.

Some of us have a legacy of fitness, and others start panting when walking more than ten steps. It doesn't matter which group you belong to; by the end of this book, you can attain a fitness level that will add joy to your senior years.

When I was young, I had a group of school friends. Some of them excelled in sports, while others were just not interested in getting all sweaty. Luckily, I belonged to the fitness group, but only just. I wasn't interested in playing for the glory of my school, but I did enjoy a game of tennis, and the swimming pool attracted me as well—but not enough to make the team. I was proud of my flexibility. I could touch my toes and do sit-ups galore.

Then came my 20s! I had a job and a social group that did not see the importance of exercise. It was also challenging to fit an exercise routine into my busy lifestyle. Soon, marriage and children entered my life—did you know that a parent must be fit? Running after the little tykes and helping them become fit enough to participate in the sport of their choice helped me get back on the fitness track. It didn't take too long to get back to my previous level of fitness. However, when the children grew up and left the nest, the couch became my favorite piece of furniture until a doctor's visit put fear in my heart.

I was now 60 with a suspected heart condition, raised blood pressure, and on the edge of type 2 diabetes. I had to get fit quickly. But that didn't happen easily. It took much longer for my creaking muscles and joints to respond.

I delved into research and finally regained my fitness—not as much as when I was young, but impressive for my age. You have the results of that research in your hand now.

AGING ISSUES

One of the worst issues of aging is that your balance suffers. You might have walked on the narrowest ledge when you were young; now, even a small incline can make you lose balance. You can educate your brain and body to help get your balance back.

Balance problems are serious. They can lead to problems getting around in your home or outside. Any quick movements, like suddenly looking over your shoulder, can result in a balance issue that may make you fall. As you age, falling becomes a real threat due to loss of balance, but there are many great exercises to help you remain upright.

You may feel that balance problems are interfering with your quality of life and that you begin to rely on others to help you along. You want to remain independent, but it is increasingly difficult. You start growing concerned about the increased risk of falls and injuries due to decreased balance and stability. The fear of falling can have profound effects on your confidence and overall well-being.

This stage of life that you have reached comes with many new problems. The first problem you have to deal with is what to do with the extra time that retirement brings. You may have lost your life partner, and physical limitations can contribute to feelings of isolation. Being physically fit and able opens opportunities for social interaction and engagement.

FALLS

While the loss of balance can be irritating, it also comes with the propensity to fall, and falls can be very serious for seniors. If you have had one fall, you are a likely candidate to fall again, so it's best to bite the bullet and use the exercises in the book to help you.

The World Health Organization (2021) states that

- Falls are a leading cause of hospitalization in the elderly. It is estimated that there are 684,000 fatal falls per annum.
- 38 million falls worldwide result in some form of disability.

The incidence of falls increases as we get older:

- Aging severely impacts our balance.
- Our muscles lose some of their strength and tone.
- If our eyesight is bad, we may trip by, for example, not seeing the height of a curb.
- A rapid head movement—up, down, or sideways—can induce dizziness, which could lead to a fall.
- Lack of concentration due to multitasking and missing hazards on the ground.

(World Health Organization, 2021)

A significant number of falls result in an injury. Injuries can vary from bruises to fractures and can affect almost any limb. The most common injuries involve the wrist—you put your hand down to try to break the fall—the lower arm bones (the radius and the ulna), your ankle, or a leg, or you end up fracturing a hip. You may connect with furniture as you go down. Striking your head could result in concussion or even death.

When you fall, you may find it challenging to get up without assistance. I once fell in my garden and couldn't get up as there was nothing near me that I could grab onto. I crawled to my car and managed to pull myself up, holding onto the door handles. My legs shook, and I was in a state of shock. Since then, I have assessed any walking route that I might take and taken my trusty walking stick with me. It is a good idea to keep your cell phone on your person 24/7. Some companies even offer you protection when you need it. You can wear a bracelet or a necklace that has a direct link to the company, and they alert an ambulance or a medical person who is in your vicinity. Some retirement homes have a similar system and require you to wear the unit all the time.

CHRONIC CONDITIONS

As we age, most of us have at least one chronic disease, such as unstable blood pressure, heart arrhythmia, or Type 2 diabetes. The more health conditions you have, the more likely a candidate you are for a fall, but fortunately, the exercises in this book will help you maintain balance and keep you away from falling.

CHANGES

As we age, our bodies undergo some changes, and if you haven't kept fit, you are asking to take a tumble. Keeping your thighs strong will help you get up after a fall. If you have had one fall, you will probably develop a fear of falling again. I understand your fear, but I can tell you that fear will decrease as you move through this book.

Bones become more brittle, and joints become stiffer, while muscles lose their flexibility. The exercises in this book will help counteract the effects of aging. Being physically fit and able brings a better quality of life and opens opportunities for social interaction and engagement.

HOW THIS BOOK CAN HELP

As someone who has gone through them, I understand the problems that come with aging, and this book will teach you tips and tricks to help you as you age.

Benefits you can experience:

- You will be introduced to "Balanced Living."
- I will show you how you can integrate exercise into your everyday life.

- We will look at exercises for both active and sedentary seniors.
- We will go through the do's and don'ts during exercise

Expected results:

- better balance, flexibility, and strength.
- Independence.
- the confidence to enjoy your mobility and vitality.
- taking part in outings with family and friends.
- While you can't turn the clock back, you will start to feel young again.

ABOUT THE AUTHOR

The author, an 85-year-old, has a deep interest in physical activities like biking and swimming and completed a century ride and several marathons.

One day, he was startled to realize that he was unknowingly holding on to things while he was getting dressed. It was so insidious that he was not even aware that he needed to work on strength and balance exercises as well. This gave him the motivation to share his experiences.

He is passionate about enabling himself and others to enjoy a high quality of life. He is a dedicated researcher and practitioner who is focused on retaining the ability to stay active every day, even in old age.

He firmly believes that lack of strength and balance heavily contributes to poor quality of life. A good quality of life, keeping our muscles toned and strong, keeps us out of nursing homes and hospitals, and helps us avoid poor balance, which leads to falls.

He adopted the concept of the "Balanced Living" framework, which sets this book apart from other books in the same genre. This new concept will help readers achieve better balance, strength, and fitness.

CHAPTER 1

UNDERSTANDING THE IMPORTANCE OF BALANCE AND FLEXIBILITY

This book deals with balance, but how do you interpret the word "balance?" Most people think about physical balance, and they would be almost right as physical balance is important, but there are many other interpretations of the word:

- **Mental balance:** Mental balance will help you handle your emotions constructively and not allow them to get the better of you. It helps us respond to issues positively and deal with interpersonal situations with care.
- **Emotional balance:** When you have attained mental balance, your emotional balance will fall into place. When you are emotionally balanced, you will remain calm and in control no matter what life throws at you.
- **Work balance:** Many of us will give our all to our work, staying behind to finish a task, no matter how long it takes. You give your all to your work and then arrive home too tired for family time. Our lives cannot just be work. We need a bit of time to play as well.

- **Physical balance:** This means that you can stay upright no
  matter what the situation is. You have control of your
  posture and can maintain physical stability.

Whenever I think of balance, I think of Lady Justice holding the
scales of justice. The scales are perfectly weighted, and that's what
we should try to achieve in all aspects of our lives. This book will
deal with two states of balance:

1. Balance for physical vigor and independence, even in
   old age
2. Balance in daily life as a whole

THE ROLE OF BALANCE AND FLEXIBILITY IN GRACEFUL AGING

Now we know that there are many interpretations for the word
"balance." As we are primarily concerned with aging in this book,
we will mainly be looking at physical balance.

Benefits of Balance in Older Adults

Good physical balance helps enhance your quality of life. You can
bend down to retrieve your golf ball. You can dance with or
without a partner. You can walk and run and play tennis or bowl.
There are other advantages for a senior to have good balance:

- **Developing better coordination:** Coordination is the
  ability to move at least two body parts at the same time.
  Balance helps you to achieve coordination and enables you
  to be in perfect control of all your bodily movements.

- **Improving your mobility:** Mobility is being able to move from place to place, over varying surfaces, and under various conditions. When you improve your balance, your mobility improves. You will be able to change directions and handle various physical activities more effectively and rapidly.
- **Preventing injury and avoiding fall risks:** Falling is a distinct possibility among seniors. When you have achieved balance, you are less susceptible to falls which means that if you are balanced and you trip, your fall will be a lot calmer, and you are less susceptible to injury.
- **Developing a faster reaction time:** A balanced body can recover more quickly from tripping over an obstacle. Balance will also help you in a crowded situation where people are nudging you as they pass by. When you are balanced, you can anticipate the presence of others and respond when presented with obstacles. You can also recover from imbalance after a sudden movement.

WHAT IS FLEXIBILITY?

Flexibility has many meanings. In work, flexibility means that you can assist in many areas, or you can be flexible about when a meeting will be held. But the flexibility I want to talk about is being flexible in your body.

As you age, your muscles and joints could show a lack of flexibility, particularly if you haven't kept up a fitness regime. Flexibility indicates that your joints and muscles can take a position and hold it without feeling pain.

Benefits of Flexibility in Older Adults

There are many reasons for seniors to keep flexible:

- If you are physically flexible, anything you need to do will be much easier.
- Your chances of injury increase as you age, but if you are flexible, your chances of injury decrease phenomenally. The possibility of muscle strains and bone fractures decreases.
- You can control chronic pain more easily, and it could possibly become a thing of the past.
- Your posture will be better. Stretching can help you attain good posture, and the risk of developing the dreaded hunch that is seen in many old people decreases.
- Your muscles and joints will function better as your flexibility improves.

SYNERGY BETWEEN BALANCE AND FLEXIBILITY

When we exercise, we need to pay attention to endurance, strength, balance, and flexibility exercises to gain the utmost benefit from our fitness routine.

Endurance

Endurance—or aerobic—exercises are good for your heart, lungs, and circulatory system. You do not have to go to a gym for endurance exercises. See if you can find something in the following list that you will enjoy—remember if exercise is a drag you won't stick with it.

- Walking—and by that, we do not mean strolling. A brisk walk will get the circulation going.
- Mowing the lawn. Ditch that lawnmower that you can sit on and get into the hand-operated ones.
- Dancing. You can choose ballroom, Latin, or even line dancing. Salsa dancing has also become very popular.
- Swimming is a good workout. The water makes you buoyant so that you do not put too much stress on an injury. Your entire body will get a workout as your arms and legs engage your torso as well.
- Riding a bicycle. Be aware of safety rules. Wear bright colors, wear a helmet, and ride with the traffic.
- Take up a hobby like tennis, badminton, volleyball, or squash (racket ball). (National Institute on Aging, 2020)

Before you start an endurance session, make sure that your muscles are warm. Cold muscles are prone to injury. You need a warm-up and a cool-down. Also, make sure to stay hydrated.

As we age, our muscles deteriorate, causing many problems, with balance being a major one. Strengthening our muscles reduces balance issues, and if our balance is good, we minimize the prospect of falling. The most important muscles that keep you upright are the calves, thighs, and hips. So, make sure to include exercises that strengthen these muscles.

You can add benefits if you use either weights or resistance during your training. When you start using weights, start with the lightest ones, as you need to build up your strength. With resistance training, you can buy lightweight bands to start.

If you follow the advice and instructions in this section, you will be rewarded with better balance, which, as we know, means that you will minimize the risk of falls.

BENEFITS BEYOND PHYSICAL HEALTH

You are working toward regaining your health physically, mentally, and spiritually. Here are some more benefits that we get from exercise beyond physical health.

- **Stress reducer:** Exercise helps release endorphins, which in turn relieve stress. It can also help reduce pain and free up the muscles, allowing for easier movement. People with better balance and flexibility are often less stressed.
- **Rejuvenation:** Your posture will improve as specific exercises can address the affected muscles. Flexibility and balance will help you move. As your muscles improve, your stability and balance will improve, giving you more confidence in yourself and your abilities. As you move with this new confidence, you will present yourself as younger.
- **Better brain and cognitive function:** As your balance improves, you will be encouraged to participate in harder and more challenging activities. These will require concentration and mindfulness. Your neural pathways will strengthen, and you will find it easier to concentrate. That concentration will improve your brain's cognitive ability.
- **Improved quality of life:** Your stress has been reduced, you look, feel, and act younger, your thought processes are improved, and your bodily movements are easier. All of this gives you more confidence to mingle with people who have the same interests as you. As you go out and about more, your spirits will be uplifted, and you will have an aura of happiness and satisfaction.

What if You Refrain from Exercise?

Most of us have a picture of what our retirement will be like, but few of us will picture ourselves in a gym doing push-ups. When we were working, we were active, and maybe we were hoping to become couch potatoes in retirement. If you follow this dream, you stand to lose more than you win.

- **Stress:** As stress builds up in your body it will affect your heart rate, blood pressure, and respiration negatively. Higher blood pressure will make you unstable and more prone to losing your balance.
- **Posture:** With no exercise, you can develop the dowager's hump more quickly. The dowager's hump—kyphosis—can develop in both sexes, although it does seem to be more common in women. It is found in the upper back, and the back curves towards the neck, which causes your head to protrude forward. Your shoulders become rounded. Your body is now in an imbalanced position, which can lead to loss of balance and then a fall.
- **Brain:** Exercise is also necessary to keep your brain and neurons healthy.
- **Quality of life:** A sedentary lifestyle feeds on itself. Making excuses to avoid exercise becomes a habit, and it is hard to break. Your muscles will lose tone, and falling becomes a definite problem.

BALANCE LOSS: INSIGHTS BEYOND THE OBVIOUS

If you suffer from loss of balance, you will feel dizzy, and with the dizziness comes instability. You may also feel nauseous. The room may appear to be rotating, and you may also feel that you are moving even if you are stationary. There are many contributing factors to the loss of balance.

Loss of balance is common with aging and is a normal part of it. As we age, we experience changes in many aspects of our lives. These changes can be the result of medication that you are taking, or the symptoms being treated can cause balance problems in themselves. Several more conditions cause imbalance:

- Meniere's disease affects the inner ear. Disruptions in the inner ear cause dizziness and loss of balance.
- Issues with your eyes can cause a loss of balance.
- Benign Paroxysmal Positional Vertigo (BPPV) is a fairly common condition among seniors that causes dizziness and/or vertigo. It usually occurs when one's head position changes, like getting up from lying down or turning one's head quickly, as may happen if someone has called out to them.
- Labyrinthitis is a virus that infects the inner ear—the part that is responsible for keeping you upright.
- Age is something we can't control, and hearing deterioration tends to happen so slowly that you adapt, usually by learning to lipread. The deterioration also affects the inner ear, which affects your balance.
- Overuse of alcohol affects your balance, so it is wise to cut down or quit.

- Some chronic conditions could disrupt the function of the inner ear, such as:

  - cardiovascular problems
  - neurological problems
  - Arthritis
  - incorrect diet

Loss of balance can occur at any time, but the number of cases escalates as we age. If you feel that you might have a balance problem, compare your symptoms with the established symptoms of loss of balance.

- vertigo
- falling—or feeling as though you are going to fall.
- Uncertainty of steps while walking—the lack of balance could cause you to meander while trying to walk straight.
- feeling faint and lightheaded or actually fainting
- feeling confused or disorientated
- blurred vision
- experiencing an anxiety or panic attack
- experiencing nausea
- experiencing a change in your heart's rhythm (National Institute on Aging, 2022)

FALL RISKS IN OLDER ADULTS

To reduce our risk of falling, we also need to look at what has caused us to fall. We are masters of our homes, and it is up to us to ensure that our homes and surroundings are free from items that may trip us up. Things to look for are loose rugs, clutter on the floor, insufficient lighting, and other tripping hazards.

You could be at risk of falling if your balance is questionable and your legs are unstable. These two conditions leave you a prime candidate for a fall, but they are not the only conditions. It is sad to note that if you had a fall, you are likely to have another one—but there are things you can do to help you stay upright. Use the following list as a checklist to see where you can improve (CDC, 2023):

- Do you hold onto various pieces of furniture as you move around the house? This is fine but it is a signal that your balance is becoming a problem.
- Do you use a walking aid? Like a walking stick or a walker. This is acceptable, but again, it illustrates that you have balance problems.
- Do you struggle to get up from a chair and use your hands to help you? If so, you need to exercise your thighs and calves.
- Can you step up—or down—at a curb? If not, calf and thigh exercises will help.
- Have you gotten your vitamin D levels checked? This is not usually done when you have your yearly checkup, so you need to ask the doctor to check this. It can be rectified by increasing your time in the sun or by taking a vitamin D supplement.
- Are you taking sleep-inducing medications? Ask your doctor if he can prescribe an alternate medication that does not cause sleepiness.

If you have eye trouble it may affect your balance. If you wear bifocals or multifocal glasses, you may be a bit disoriented and lose balance. Remember to check your vision at least once every two years. As you get older, your eyesight may deteriorate quicker, and you may need to go to the optician more often.

Every new mother wants to baby-proof their home, well now is the time for you to safety-proof your home! Check on loose rugs and make sure that they do not curl up on the edges as that is a fall waiting to happen. If you have a staircase, get handrails on both sides. Install grab bars in the bathroom—there should be one in the shower and one by the toilet. Darkness isn't your friend— apologies to Simon and Garfunkel. Your home needs to be well lit: Install more lights in dark areas. Use stronger globes in your light fittings.

Fall Risk Statistics

Some fall risk statistics for older adults (CDC, 2021):

- 20% of falls will need a hospital visit, particularly if you hit your head. You may also break a bone.
- If you have a fall that requires you to visit the Emergency Room, you are just 1 in 3 million this year.
- Head and hip injuries account for 800,000 hospital patients.
- Hips injured by a fall (usually a sideways fall) account for 95% of hip injuries.

Fall Risk Checklist

Go through this checklist to see if you are at risk of falling. The first column in the table is for a yes or no answer. In the end, you need to have more no's than yeses to be stable when moving around. But do not despair, this book will help you gain stability. Do the test now and repeat it after you have followed the recommended exercises in this book. (This table has been adapted from a 2023 brochure from the CDC).

Y/N	Description
	I have fallen at least once in this year.
	I use a mobility aid—such as a walking stick or a walker.
	I am unsteady when I walk.
	I hold onto the furniture as I walk around my home.
	I need help getting out of a chair. I usually use my hands.
	I need help when I climb onto or off the curb.
	One of my medicines makes me drowsy.

THE RIGHT BALANCE OF FREQUENCY AND INTENSITY

When you choose which form of exercise suits you, make sure that it addresses balance, fitness, and strength. A lack of strength in your legs can contribute to your imbalance.

Remember that you need to enjoy the type of exercise if you do not want it to become a drag.

The target time to spend on your exercise is 150 minutes per week, but in the beginning, you will be spending a lot less time as you work to improve your fitness. The 150 minutes is split into 30 minutes a day for five days of the week. Again, this is the target time, but you need to build up to it. The two rest days can be the weekend, or you could do three exercise days, one day of rest, then two exercise days, and then enjoy the other day of rest. In the beginning, 10 to 15 minutes a day is quite acceptable.

The 150 minutes of exercise allow you to do moderately intensive exercise. If you prefer to exercise vigorously, you can cut the time down to 75 minutes per week, which equals 15 minutes per day.

You can also mix and match: Do three days of vigorous exercise and two days of moderate exercise. Another way you can mix and match is to have a mixture of moderate and intense exercises on the same day. Whatever you choose, make sure you enjoy it.

Every exercise day should include one or more balanced exercises. On two of the days, you must include exercises that strengthen your body, particularly the legs.

Some examples of exercise formats (CDC, 2019):

- Mowing the lawn really gets your motor running. If at the end, you are breathless and have an elevated heartbeat, it qualifies as a strenuous workout.
- The next time you get into your car to go to the corner shop, why not walk instead? Of course, you need to put safety first. Try to walk in a group. That walk could qualify as a moderate exercise if you stroll there or a strenuous exercise if you run.
- Join a dance class, either ballroom, Latin, or line dancing. Sometimes, dancing can be quite strenuous.
- Join a Yoga or tai chi class for moderate exercise.
- Go for a hike. If you are a beginner, choose flat terrain. If you are experienced, then the more hills the better.
- If walking is not your thing, then go for a bicycle ride. A stationary bike is also a good alternative.
- If you like swimming, you can join a water aerobics class.

WILL HEALTH ISSUES INTERFERE WITH MY EXERCISE PROGRESS?

It is never too late to start an exercise program. Most people are fine with entering a program, but if you are a bit worried about your present condition, see if the answer to your problem is here.

Before starting any exercise program, it is wise to visit your doctor and discuss your health condition and the type of exercise that appeals to you.

Chronic Conditions and Exercising

So, what are chronic conditions? Asthma, irregular heartbeat, arthritis, blood pressure problems, and diabetes are all considered to be chronic.

- **Heart issues (like a heart attack):** Very soon after suffering the attack or the operation, you can start walking. Slowly does it. To start, you will take a gentle stroll and keep the distance short. The idea is to get back to exercising slowly. Gradually increase the speed of your step until you are walking—rather than strolling. Once you are comfortable walking, increase the distance slowly. Just remember your walk will take you away from home, and you need to get back, so reserve some energy for the return trip.
- **A stroke:** After a stroke, your first exercises should be done seated and should target a limb that has been affected by the stroke as well as your healthy limbs. When you have built up strength doing seated exercises, you can progress to standing exercises.
- **Diabetes:** Many studies have proved that exercise helps our bodies cope with the onslaught of diabetes (CDC, 2020a).
- **Asthma (or other breathing problem):** Start slowly, preferably doing seated exercises, building up to walking short distances. As your lungs begin to adjust, you can increase the time and the strength of your exercise program.

- **Arthritis:** The affected limbs will do well if you limit the session to slow strength-building exercises. Walking and water aerobics are good places to start.

Keep a record of your progress. The first entry should be after a week and the next one after a month. When you reach the three-month mark, you will be surprised at how well you are doing.

Exercise is very important if you have any form of disability. Some of the exercises can be done as explained, and most can be adjusted to help.

THINGS TO REMEMBER BEFORE EXERCISING

Difficulty Levels

In the previous section, I mentioned taking things slowly at the start. I would like to expand on that thought. Have a chat with your medical advisor before rushing into an exercise program.

- **Beginner:** Start here if you haven't exercised for a while or if you have been a couch potato, but you know that you have to start exercising. Start here as well If you have a disability or a chronic condition.
- **Intermediate:** Once you have been doing the beginner program for two or three weeks and you are feeling good then it is time to step it up. You can check with your medical advisor if you wish.
- **Advanced:** You need to stick to the intermediate program for two to three weeks. If your body has adapted to all the exercises, it is time to move on to the advanced level. You may like to brag when you visit your medical advisor.

- **Expert Status:** If you are very healthy and have no adverse ailments, you can transfer to expert status. Expert status implies that you are an active adult and that your bragging rights belong to you.

Basic Muscle Anatomy

MUSCULAR SYSTEM

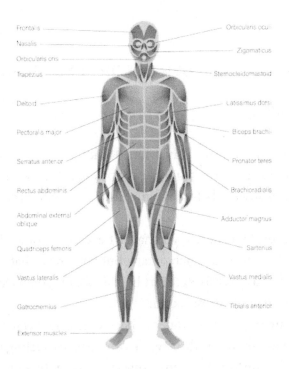

Image by Freepik

At one time—and not so long ago—we believed that it was normal to be incapacitated as you age. But now the experts acknowledge that we can remain fit for the rest of our days if we are willing to put in the effort. So, it is time to get active.

Here are the main muscle groups we target through exercise:

- **Glutes:** Basically, we are talking about the muscles in your bottom. These muscles are powerful as they sit at the seat of your back muscles. If they are strong, back problems will lessen. Strong glutes will also have an impact on your knees.
- **Back muscles:** These extend from the glutes up to the neck. If these are weak you may have chronic pain and even develop a dowager hump—as discussed earlier. Everything we do places a strain on these muscles so we need to incorporate exercises that will strengthen them.
- **Chest muscles:** These muscles are responsible for giving strength to your arms.
- **Shoulder muscles:** The shoulder muscles take up the job that the chest muscles started. These muscles are used whenever you work on the other areas of your body. They extend from the front to the sides and towards the back.
- **Quadriceps:** These are your thigh muscles. They are very important as they control most of your movements as well as allow you to stand from a seated position. Many people just concentrate on the upper body, but it is essential to include exercises that strengthen your thighs.
- **Hamstrings:** When you forget about your hamstrings, you are potentially inviting tears in your other muscle groups. Tight hamstrings stop you from being able to touch your toes. While you might think that's fine, I don't need to touch my toes, healthy, stretched hamstrings will complement all the other muscle groups in attaining fitness.
- **Calves:** These are probably the most used muscles in your body. You use them when you walk, run, jump, and use your feet.

- **Triceps:** These are the long muscles at the back of your arms. They stabilize the shoulder muscles.
- **Biceps:** These are found in the upper arm and help to stabilize the shoulders.
- **Abs:** These are a band of muscles that extend from your tummy region to the back. They support the upper body and strength. Strength in these muscles—which form your core—helps you stay upright. Strength in your core helps you stand up from a seated position without using your arms and to stand up straight.
- **Forearms:** These muscles help you grip anything, grab onto, and carry heavy items.

SEGUE

This chapter has laid the foundation for your exercise program. We discussed the importance of balance. Balance will allow you to exercise better, while a lack of balance is one of the most likely causes of falls among seniors.

We have now established a basis for the following chapters in the book, where we will discuss specific exercises. The next chapter is called "Essential and Quick Fitness Routine #1: Split Squats."

CHAPTER 2
ESSENTIAL AND QUICK FITNESS ROUTINE #1: SPLIT SQUATS

Split Squat

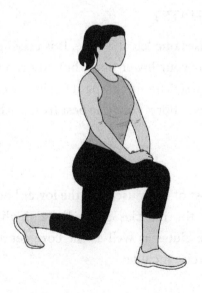

N ow we get to the exciting part—the part where you learn exercises to help you. I will explain how to do each exercise in small, easy-to-follow steps.

I know you are battling with balance; otherwise, this book would not have found a home with you. As you do this exercise, you will gradually become more supple, and your balance problems will diminish. You will find that your lower body, in particular, your leg muscles, will gain strength and mobility. If you have back problems, you will find relief.

Does this sound familiar? You wake up in the morning, your back is sore, your legs feel shaky, and you really want to stay in bed. Commit yourself to an exercise routine and check in with yourself in three months to see if that has changed—are you now keen and eager to start the day?

WHY SPLIT SQUATS?

A split squat exercises one leg at a time. It is classified as an intermediate exercise for your lower body, but you can start small and gradually build yourself up. It can be described as a combination of squats and lunges— borrowing the best from each exercise.

Benefits

Split squats use most of the muscles of the lower body and exercise the entire leg. All the muscles around the thigh including the hamstrings and the glutes as well as the core get a workout. The benefits of this exercise include:

- Strength is improved.
- Joints become more flexible, and mobility is increased.
- Back pain decreases.
- Balance improves.

What to Expect After Doing This Exercise Regularly

The first time that you do this exercise, you will probably become aware that one side of your body is stronger than the other. This is not something weird, we all are either right-handed or left-handed. So why can the same not be true of your legs? It doesn't necessarily follow that if you are right-handed, you will be right-legged. By doing split squats you will quickly establish which is your weak side. If you are still a bit puzzled, stand with your feet slightly apart and take a step forward. You will automatically move the stronger leg without even thinking about it. Once you have established which is your weak side, you can perhaps add on a few extra repetitions on that side.

After a week, you will be doing the exercise with less effort, your balance will improve, and other leg exercises will become a bit easier. Your joints will be more mobile, and you will see that your muscles are a bit firmer than the week before.

After one month there will be a marked improvement in your balance. Your lower body will be stronger and more flexible.

After three months, your lower body will be the strongest it has ever been. Any backache symptoms will be less painful, and your back will be more supple. Walking will be more pleasurable as normal movements—like bending, lifting, and walking—will be stronger, easier, and less painful. You might opt to do split squats with weights.

If you are unfit and haven't exercised for a couple of years, you might want to spend a couple of weeks leading up to the split squat. You can introduce normal squats for a couple of sessions. Don't worry if you can't do a proper squat at first—go down as far as you feel comfortable. You will notice that the squat improves every time you do it.

HOW TO PROPERLY DO SPLIT SQUAT: STEP-BY-STEP GUIDE

Generally speaking, weights, resistor bands, or other physical aids will not be necessary. What is necessary is addressing your balance problems. Make sure that you have some support close by, whether it's a friend, a chair, or the wall. I suggest you have a chair close by or a friend. The friend's job will be to leave you alone unless they see that you are about to fall. The chair is there to grab onto if you start to lose balance.

Stand with your feet slightly apart. Move your right foot forward as far as is comfortable, making sure that your left heel stays in contact with the floor. Make sure your selected support is close to your right side.

As you enter the lunge, make sure that the ball of your left foot stays contact with the floor.

1. Bend your front knee as you lunge forward, keeping your posture as upright as you can.
2. As you sink into the lunge, bend your right knee. At first, you will probably only be able to bend it a bit, but that is fine. As you get better, you will be able to bend it more until it makes a right angle from the calf to the foot. If you try to bend it too much at first, you may find it difficult to

balance your body. Remember that saying, "You have to walk before you can run."

3. Bend the left knee until it touches the ground. You may not get it so low on your first few attempts, but that is fine. As you practice, your knee will get lower until it touches the floor. For now, bend the back knee as far as it is comfortable.

4. Keep your movement slow and controlled.

5. Use your right leg to straighten up. You may use your support to help you. If it is really necessary, you can get your back leg to help you, but you are aiming for the front leg to do the work.

6. Repeat the stretch on the left side.

Difficulty Levels

Once you have the basics down, you can adjust the exercise according to your level.

- **Beginner:** Do exactly as described above. You can start with three repetitions with each leg and increase gradually until you are doing ten reps with each leg. As you get better at it, your back knee will get closer to the floor. When you can achieve this, move on to the next set.
- **Intermediate:** Increase the number of repetitions. When you can do 15 reps with each leg you are ready to move on.
- **Advanced:** Increase to 20 reps and work to get your back knee to the floor.

Important Tips

Let's look at some tips that will help you get the most out of any exercise routine.

Posture is important for all exercises. Keep the upper torso firm and keep your back straight unless the exercise specifies that you bend your back. Your shoulders must be down and not scrunched up towards your ears, again, unless the exercise specifically states that you must scrunch your shoulders to your ears.

The next two points are specifically for split squats.

- Your weight should be distributed evenly so that your back foot does not support the majority of your weight. There should be enough tension on the floor so that your foot doesn't move around.
- Don't spread your legs so wide that it causes stress on the joints. The exercise should stretch the limbs but only to a comfortable point.

Balanced Living: How to Incorporate this Exercise into Daily Life

If you find yourself often saying, "I really wish I had time for exercising, but there's just no time in my schedule," then I have the solution for you: Incorporate exercises into your daily work or leisure time.

- **Morning routine:** While brushing your teeth, do at least one split squat on each leg. While waiting for the bath to fill or the shower to warm up, do a couple of split squats. This will help set a positive tone for the day.

- **TV time:** During TV commercials, instead of rushing to the fridge for a snack or a drink, stand up and do a set of split squats. This adds some movement during sedentary moments.
- **Laundry:** As you fold laundry, use the laundry room countertop or a stable surface for split squats. Do one set of split squats for every three items you deal with.
- **Taking the stairs:** Incorporate split squats while climbing stairs. Step onto a stair, perform a split squat, and repeat on the other side.

EXERCISE AND STRESS

Modern life holds stress for all of us, whether we are, students, employees, or retirees. Almost half the population does not exercise due to time constraints. A little bit of exercise can lower a person's stress levels, and it is by far the easiest and cheapest way to do so. Stress interferes with a person's ability to relax and switch off to give the body time to recover. It affects the mind, body, and spirit. Stress can contribute to many ailments like:

- Finding it hard to concentrate on the task at hand.
- Tossing and turning in bed instead of having a relaxing sleep to prepare for the day ahead.
- Eating: It might lead to over-eating or having no appetite for food.
- Stomach issues are caused by over- or under-eating.
- Worsening existing health conditions.
- Feelings of anxiety or depression.

Some ideas to help you handle your stress:

- Be in the moment. If you are watching TV focus on what you are looking at. If you have a drink in your hand, focus on sipping it. Is it hot or cold? Is it sweet? If you are in a social situation, listen to what people are saying, make eye contact. Contribute if you have something useful to say.
- Try journaling. When negativity strikes, write down what is bothering you. This will help you deal with the problems as you see them more clearly. Don't beat yourself up for all the things you perceive you did wrong. Be kind to yourself and others.
- Pay attention to what you watch on TV. Terrible things are happening in today's world. They will happen whether or not you watch footage on TV. Good mental health needs good news.
- Get into a routine. If your day is routine-driven, you don't have to stress about having time for everything. Everything will fall into place as time progresses.
- Exercise. This is what I consider to be the best stress fighter! When you exercise, you are almost forced to be in the moment. You concentrate on the movements contained in that exercise, so negativity goes out the window. The movements of the exercise will help you relax, and relaxation is a stress reliever. As you exercise, your breathing is important, and just concentrating on your breathing will help you handle stress.

SEGUE

Although this chapter is primarily to introduce you to split squats, there are also many health and well-being tips. The first tip is to help you minimize falls when waking up and getting out of bed. Falls are the number one risk for pensioners. Split squats will help build up strength in the lower body. If you are strong in the lower body, you can minimize the risk of falling.

I have taken you through split squats as a beginner. As you feel more confident as a beginner, you move on to the next stage, intermediate squats. This is followed by advanced techniques in squats, and finally, you are ready to move into the expert zone.

The next chapter deals with the next exercise on your fitness journey: Chair Raises.

CHAPTER 3
ESSENTIAL AND QUICK FITNESS ROUTINE #2: CHAIR RAISES

Chair raises

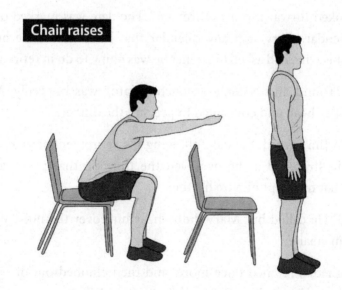

Although it is natural for us to get more sedentary as we age, it doesn't have to be the rule. We need to encourage ourselves to be as active as we were before retirement.

Life was shorter in our grandparents' days. As they aged, they became less active, and their health began to decrease. We now know that there is no rule book that says your fitness has to deteriorate once you retire. In fact, the fitter you are, the better your life will be, as your general health will be stable and improved.

THE STORY OF MARY AND JIM

Let us look at a scenario:

Jim looked forward to his retirement. The date was marked off on his calendar, diary, and any calendar that he found in the house, Mary, his wife, had asked him what he was going to do in retirement.

"Laze around and become a couch potato," was his reply. Mary shook her head and continued to prepare the dinner.

True to Jim's word, the day following his retirement started at 11 a.m. He stretched as he observed the time on that pesky alarm clock that had kept him on his toes.

"Mary!" He called but Mary didn't hear him over the noise of the vacuum cleaner.

Jim sighed, stretched once more, and then climbed out of bed to find Mary. "It shouldn't be hard," he muttered. That vacuum makes such a loud noise."

He found her in the lounge.

"Mary, your vacuuming woke me up!" he moaned.

"Jim, you know it is 11 o'clock already?"

"Yep," he answered. "What's for breakfast?"

"Breakfast?" queried Mary. "It's almost lunchtime."

"Well, that's fine. I'll have brunch!" and he tottered into the den, sprawled himself out on the couch, and switched the TV on.

This became his norm, and he didn't realize that as each lazy day dawned, he was getting more unfit, and his clothes were getting noticeably tight. The walk to the den seemed to get longer each day. But he was soon to get a nightmare of a day which would make him regret his attitude.

The day dawned bright and clear, although Jim only saw it at 11 a.m. He was pleased to experience the quiet around him. Then he thought "That's odd, why isn't Mary vacuuming?"

He crawled out of bed and went searching for Mary. He was shocked into action when he saw her lying on the floor.

"Mary! What happened?"

"I fell and now can't get up. I need help."

"Sure, old girl, I can help you," Jim said as he got into position. His first attempt was unsuccessful, as he didn't seem to have strength in his arms. After a few more unsuccessful attempts to help Mary, he shook his head and fell to the floor next to her.

"Just let me get my breath, then I'll try again," he said, but he would have to get up first, and that was not happening. There they both were—stranded on the floor and unable to get up by themselves or with each other's help. Jim crawled to the phone and phoned their daughter. When his distress call was over, he tried to pull himself up using the telephone table, but his legs were just not strong enough. He crawled back to Mary to wait for their daughter to rescue them.

When they were finally up and about sitting with their daughter, they had to listen to her gentle scolding.

"Mom and Dad, this was not good. What if I hadn't been able to get to you until tonight? Dad, you have let yourself go, and Mom, housework may feel as if it keeps you fit, but you need more. Both of you need to join a fitness class."

Now let's look at Jim and Mary three months down the road. Their fitness class concentrates on movements that help tone up their lower body. The most significant exercise was chair raises which strengthen their thighs, abs, back, and glutes. Getting up and down now was a cinch.

BENEFITS OF CHAIR RAISES

When you need to stand up from a seated position, many muscles come into play. You need to have strength in all the muscles from your diaphragm to your calves. Chair raises will help strengthen those muscles.

The first few chair raises will be difficult but as your muscles get toned, it will get easier and easier. Before you start your exercise program you probably have to use your arms to help you get up from a chair. So set yourself an aim to be able to get up from a chair with no effort.

It will be a good idea, before you start your full exercise program, to test how many times you can stand up and then seat yourself in a 30-second test. This test will form a baseline that can be compared with another test at one week, then at one month, and then at three months, and so forth.

The Test   ✓

You need a good stable chair with no arms and a timer—most cell phones have a timer and a stopwatch. It will be easier for the test if you have someone to help with doing the 30-second countdown, while you do the following steps:

1. Sit in the chair with your arms crossed in front of your chest—hands to your shoulders.
2. Your feet should be shoulder-width apart. One foot can be slightly in front of the other foot.
3. The timer starts when you start on your first attempt to stand up.
4. Stand up fully—if you can.
5. Lower to sit on the chair, making sure you are fully seated.
6. Start the next stand-up.

Your score is how many times you can do it in 30 seconds. When I started, my score was zero, but I have built up to a very satisfying 15. If you are battling to get up from a chair or picking up a heavy packet of groceries, you need to strengthen your muscles. There are quite a few benefits to doing chair raisers:

- You will strengthen your hips, thighs, buttocks, abs, and lower back muscles.
- You will notice a positive change in your posture.

Why Is This Routine Essential?

As with any exercise, this one helps you burn calories, but more importantly, it strengthens all muscles in the mid-to-lower body. As your abs get stronger, you will notice that your posture has improved. When seniors have bad posture, they look years older than their actual age. The reverse is also true: Good posture seems to help you shed years from your biological age. Better posture will also help with your balance.

This routine also improves your circulation which leads to better heart health. Improved circulation will also help combat any chronic conditions you may have. Your general health will be better, which will help you to fight infections like a cold or flu.

Changes You Can Expect

As you go through your exercise plan you will notice some changes and improvements. You can expect the following changes if you are exercising at least five days a week.

After one week:

You should notice a couple of changes at the end of a week's exercise.

- Your joint mobility will be better.
- Your thighs will get stronger.

You will notice that it is easier to go from sitting to standing and that your balance improves while walking.

After one month:

The excitement of the changes after only one week will give you the motivation to continue, and as the days go by, you will notice the following improvements:

- Your lower body will be much stronger, giving you the strength to stand up unassisted.
- Your balance will be much improved, giving you the confidence to "strut your stuff."

After three months:

You will be surprised at how much you have generally improved:

- Your core will be much stronger and more flexible.
- Your overall strength will be improved.
- You will notice an improvement in your thigh muscles.

All of these improvements will protect you from falls as your strength, and your balance will be much improved.

Goals

You can use the following tables to see how you are doing. The first table is for women, and the second one is for men. Find your age group in the first column. While you are still starting up, the goals may seem unattainable. You must try to bring your repetitions to the average column at least. The second column gives your range if you are less than average. The third column is considered average—aim for this figure first. The last column cheers you on as it is above average.

Goals for Women

Age	Below Average (Less than)	Average	Above average (More than)
60 to 64	12	12 to 17	17
65 to 69	11	11 to 16	16
70 to 74	10	10 to 15	15
75 to 79	10	10 to 15	15
80 to 84	9	9 to 14	14
85 to 89	8	8 to 13	13
90 to 94	4	4 to 11	11

Goals for Men

Age	Below Average (Less than)	Average	Above average (More than)
60 to 64	14	14 to 19	19
65 to 69	12	12 to 18	18
70 to 74	12	12 to 17	17
75 to 79	11	11 to 17	17
80 to 84	10	10 to 15	15
85 to 89	8	8 to 14	14
90 to 94	7	7 to 12	12

General Tips

Before you start exercising, I would like to give you some tips:

- Dress in something comfortable and loose.
- Keep some water close by.
- When starting a new exercise start with just a couple of reps.
- If the exercise is uncomfortable or very hard, you may not have the stamina to do it. Leave it for a week or so before trying it again.
- You need a chair for this exercise and for some of the others in this book. It must be stable, so a chair with wheels is not a good idea. It preferably should not have arms.
- When you sit on the chair make sure that your feet can rest on the floor with your knees naturally bent.

CHAIR RAISES

Equipment: Your chair with a straight back without armrests (seat 17" high).

Instructions:

1. Sit comfortably on the chair. Make sure that you are in the middle of the seat with your legs comfortably flat on the floor.
2. Cross your arms in front of your chest. Your left hand is close to your right shoulder and your right hand is close to your left shoulder.
3. Make sure that your back is kept as straight as possible and keep your arms against your chest.

4. Rise to a standing position.
5. Sit back down on the chair ready for your next chair raise.

Difficulty Levels

Some of us will be absolute beginners and others may be fit so I will explain how everyone can benefit from this exercise.

- **Beginner:** As explained above. Try to do at least three reps on the first day and then add more when three becomes easy.
- **Intermediate:** For this level, only your arms will change. Instead of holding your arms to your body, you will stretch them out in front of you.
- **Advanced:** Keep your arms straight ahead and increase the reps. Try to get as many reps as is indicated in the table for your gender and age group.
- **Expert:** For this level, we need to speed things up. So that you only sit for a split second and revert to sitting as quickly as you can when you stand.

FOCUS DURING EXERCISE

Exercise will help you cope with all the stress and health conditions that come with retirement. You should notice an improvement in your blood pressure and your sleep quality. Exercise will also lessen the chances of developing dementia, heart issues, and strokes.

When you are exercising, be in the moment by concentrating on the exercise as well as your breathing.

Use your breath to guide you through the chair rise. Take a big breath and as you exhale, stand up. On the next inhale sit down. And so, the exercise continues—sit down on the inhale and stand up on the exhale.

Make sure that you are in control, particularly when you sit down. Don't just flop down. All your movements must be done slowly and with control. Keep your posture upright throughout. It is very tempting to use your shoulders and back to help you up. Your thighs, hips, and abs should be engaged to get up and sit down again.

BALANCED LIVING

Sometimes your day is so busy that you battle to find the time for your exercise session. As long as this is not just an excuse, it is possible to find those minutes during the day when you can exercise.

How to incorporate this exercise into daily life:

- When you wake up in the morning get to your chair and do a few chair raises.
- Before having a meal, you can spend a few minutes doing some chair raises.
- When you switch the kettle on instead of standing mindlessly in front of it waiting for it to boil, get to your chair for some chair raises.
- If you are watching a show on the TV, there will be commercial breaks. Use them to get a few chair raises under your belt.
- If you are watching a show on Netflix or other streaming companies, reward yourself by doing some chair raises before you watch your program.

SEGUE

You now have two exercises in your fitness armory. Both exercises work the lower body as well as your posture and your balance.

You can decide if you want to take the test before starting the exercise or not. However, the purpose of doing the test is to demonstrate your fitness level, so it is beneficial to take it every month to track your improvement.

As you move through your exercise program, you will start to see an improvement in your fitness and stability. Keep your goals in sight and work hard to achieve them.

Remember to be in the moment when you exercise. Think of the muscles you are using. You can play music while you exercise but preferably songs without vocals as you could get distracted and start to sing along.

When you are planning your day make sure that you allocate some time for your exercise

CHAPTER 4
ESSENTIAL AND QUICK FITNESS ROUTINE #3: SINGLE LEG STANCE

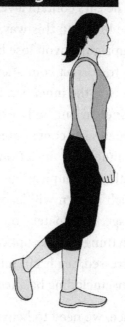

Single Leg Stance

W e all know that we are either right-handed or left-handed, but did you know we also have a dominant leg? This dominant leg does more work than the other one. It might be the left or the right. If you don't know which one is dominant, stand with your feet together and decide to start walking. The dominant leg will usually move first.

This chapter deals with exercising each leg separately to force the lazy leg to get stronger. This exercise also challenges your balance.

BALANCE AND FALLS

As we get older balance becomes an issue. Our bodies are marvelous, every part of our body has functions that either depend on or help another part. Who would have thought that balance is dictated by the ears? The ears contain a vestibular system that is in direct contact with the brain. In this way, the brain and ear work together to keep you upright. If you lose balance the brain acts on the message and helps to correct your stance so that you don't fall. The vestibular section is in the inner ear. It consists of many small parts—the smallest bones in our body exist in the inner ear. The inner ear has cilia which also contributes to balance and can be damaged due to an inner ear infection like labyrinthitis. The damage interferes with communication with the brain and can lead to imbalance which in turn will lead to falls. The cells in the ear also die off as we age. Fortunately, our brain is wired to adjust to this damage, but anything can disrupt communication causing a fall. If you are ill or stressed, the brain must deal with that as well as all its other functions, including balance.

To improve our balance, we need to help the brain by doing exercises like single-leg stance. As your brain gets used to the movements, it can draw on the knowledge and will try to keep you upright. You can help your brain's conditioning by doing exercises that are selected specifically to help with balance.

Balance Techniques

Any sudden head movement could cause you to lose balance. Let's say you are walking—with or without a mobility aid—and a friend calls to you. You turn quickly in their direction and down you go. What would have been preferable is to slowly turn your whole body in the direction of their voice.

If you drop something and swoop down to pick it up, you will go down. You will feel a bit dizzy as your brain tries to adjust to the movement. It will be better if you hold onto something as you slowly drop, bend your knees, and drop your body as low as is needed to grab the item.

Watch where you walk. An uneven surface may cause you to lose balance. If you know you are going to encounter an uneven surface, it will help if you wear sturdy shoes and use a mobility aid like a walking stick or a walker.

Slow down, particularly if your legs lack strength. The faster you go the less in control you will be.

You Are in Control

The exercise in this chapter will help strengthen your standing leg. The strength in your legs will support your brain in keeping you upright and balanced. Your improved balance will help keep you stable while walking or doing chores. You will also notice the difference when your head moves up or down or side to side.

After a few exercise sessions, you might notice an improvement when you are just walking through the house, reaching up to a top shelf, or bending down to pick up something.

WHY IS THIS ROUTINE ESSENTIAL?

Our balance is getting worse: Falls are the second biggest cause of accidental deaths worldwide, and falls are due to balance issues (Mosley, 2023). Dr Michael Mosley explains the increase in falls is the result of our jobs keeping us moving, but now we spend too much time sitting in front of a computer or TV screen.

When you use your balance, your brain, eyes, ears, muscles, and joints all work together. Earlier I explained how the brain and the ears coordinate to keep you balanced, but your eyes also play an important part. If you don't believe me, just try this simple test: Stand on one leg and close your eyes. Before you try this, make sure that there is something or someone close by that you can grab onto if you wobble.

I mentioned the possibility of the "wobble" as you try to do the one-leg stand, don't stop if you do wobble. Wobbling is good (Mosley, 2023). As you lift the foot of the leg you are going to raise, you engage your brain and all the body parts previously mentioned. The brain tries to make sense of the situation and will store it for later use. If you are wobbling, your brain stores that fact and will work to try to counteract it. The brain will recognize that the wobble is not part of the exercise, but it is part of the work that it has to do in the future.

Benefits

One of the benefits of this exercise is that it engages various body parts, including your brain. Other benefits include:

- Your balance will improve the more you do the exercise.
- Your brain will get some exercise in coordination.
- Your core strength will improve.
- Your posture will improve. With an improved posture, you will appear younger than your years.
- You will also feel younger and will be prepared to try new things.
- Your confidence will improve with your balance.

You will be amazed at your improvement in many areas if you do this exercise regularly.

After one week:

Try to do this exercise at least five times a week then you will notice:

- You can achieve so much more physically as your muscles are getting toned.
- You will become more aware of how parts of your body move together. As your awareness grows, you will start to get more out of your exercise sessions.
- You will be aware of an improved balance.

After one month:

- Your balance will improve markedly. This is great because the better your balance, the less likely you are to fall.
- Your abs, thighs, and glutes will be stronger.

- If you look at how some older people walk, you will notice that many sway from side to side. If that was a problem for you it will now be straightened out.

After three months:

- Your general balance will be much improved.
- Your stamina will be much better.
- Your movements will be more fluid.
- Your posture will have improved.
- Everyday tasks will seem easier.

THE SINGLE LEG STANCE

The table below summarizes how long the various age groups should aim to keep a one-leg stance. You may not get there immediately but with practice, you may even do better than the table suggests.

Age	Eyes Open	Eyes closed
50-59 years old	37 seconds	4.8 seconds
60-69 years old	26.9 seconds	2.8 seconds
70-79 years old	18.3 seconds	2 seconds
80-99 years old	5.6 seconds	1 second

Step-by-Step Guide

It is always good, when you start exercising, to make note of how well you did the first time you tried it. This is called setting a baseline. After a week (about 5 occasions that you do the exercise) get a helper to capture your progress. You can try to capture your progress every week. It will help you stay motivated to exercise when you see how well you are doing.

Baseline Test

To achieve this, you are going to need a helper and a chair or other surface that you can grab onto if you lose balance.

1. Stand straight up with your feet comfortably together.
2. Lift one foot off the floor. Do not let it wrap around the standing leg or even rest against the leg, as this will give you a bit more stability and defeat the exercise's object.
3. If you have a helper, get them to time you on a stopwatch or the timer app that most cell phones have. They must start timing as soon as you lift your foot. It will be a bit difficult if you don't have a helper. You could still use the stopwatch app, but it might be easier if there is a clock on the wall that shows the seconds. Make a note of the number.
4. For this baseline test, you need to do each leg with your eyes open and then again with your eyes closed.

Just a tip for later: If this exercise starts to get too easy, introduce some instability! Stand on a pillow to do the exercise.

Once you have done the baseline test, you can start the exercise.

Instructions For the Exercise

Equipment: A stable chair.

Instructions:

1. Stand behind the chair and hold on with both hands.
2. Slowly lift one leg off the ground and hold the pose for at least five seconds.

3. Lower the leg to the starting position.
4. Repeat five times, trying to increase the amount of time in the pose.
5. Repeat with the other leg.

Difficulty Levels

The above exercise is for beginners. As you become more experienced you might like to bring in some variations.

- **Intermediate:** When you are feeling confident you can change to a one-hand hold on the chair.
- **Advanced:** At this stage, you will no longer hold on to the chair. You will, however, need to stand close to the chair, which is there for safety. Do the exercise described earlier but now you will do a set with your eyes open and then another set with your eyes closed.
- **Expert:** Do this extension close to a chair. One never knows when a loss of balance will strike. When you have lifted one foot rise onto the toes of the standing leg. Try it with open eyes then with closed eyes.

Further Extensions

When you have achieved the expert level, you may like to try some of these variations. While standing on one leg:

- Slowly nod your head up and down.
- Slowly shake your head to the left and right.
- Extend the raised leg to the side.
- Extend the raised leg forwards.
- Extend the raised leg to the back being careful to keep your posture upright.

- You can try different arm positions: to the side or raised.
- Stand on a pillow.

BEST PRACTICES

This is a very important exercise. We stand on two legs, but we walk on one at a time! This means we use both legs to walk, but at any time, you have one leg down and one leg up! If you are battling to walk and you find yourself shuffling along, be aware that it a) makes you appear older than you are to the people around you and b) causes your posture to suffer and makes you become round-shouldered easier which will make you feel old.

The more upright you are the better your posture will be and the more confident you will feel. When you start the one-leg raise exercise you may only manage to get your foot a few inches off the floor. That is perfectly fine, the purpose of the exercise is to strengthen the standing leg. As you progress you will find that you can lift the leg higher until your thigh is almost parallel to the floor.

If you have a balance problem, this exercise becomes even more important. The more you do it, the better your balance will be when walking.

Warm Up

Warming up is important before you start any form of exercise. Cold muscles invite injury. A warm-up can be as simple as walking or, if you wish, running for a few minutes. Both are good warm-up exercises as they involve your whole body.

Some other ideas for warming up:

- If going outside doesn't appeal to you, march on the spot or jog in place for a few minutes.
- Walking up and down a flight of stairs. Make sure that the flight of stairs has a handrail. Many seniors have lost balance climbing stairs and a fall could be disastrous.
- Stretches:
- Extend your arms up, forward, or to the sides. Do some lunges to stretch your legs.
- Do some arm circles and shoulder shrugs to warm up your upper body.
- Turn your head to the sides, stretching your neck. Then lift your head until your eyes see the ceiling. Drop your head to see the floor. Repeat the stretches a few times.

General Tips

This exercise—and many others that we will deal with—needs to be done slowly to get the full benefit of it.

Your lack of balance means you need to have firm support nearby. That support could be a person or an item of furniture. Because you will be using a chair for some of the exercises, that item can be the chair, so make sure it is stable and preferably without arms.

FINDING THE TIME

Most people nowadays lead busy lives, and some will use that as an excuse to avoid exercising. You might hear from those shirkers, "I am far too busy to do exercises." Well, I will specify some answers you could give to this excuse.

There are many times in a day when you are waiting for things when you can fit in some exercises:

- **Waiting for the kettle to boil:** You could fit in a few leg raises instead of staring mindlessly into space.
- **While brushing your teeth:** The hand basin is a sturdy piece of equipment. Hang on to it with your free hand and do some leg raises. Talk about multitasking!
- **While talking on the phone:** You could do either leg raises or chair raises.
- If you are still working, there will be many occasions where you could pinch a minute or two. For example, waiting for the photocopier—either waiting for your turn or waiting for the copies—or waiting to speak to the boss, for example.

SEGUE

Things start changing as we age. Twenty years ago, we were probably employed, and even if we did not consciously exercise, our lives were busy, and we were active. Now, it is all too easy to sit back and watch TV or a new show on Netflix. Instead of keeping ourselves active, we become couch potatoes. However, it is possible to be active in your 70s, 80s, and even 90s.

One of the problems with aging is that you start to lose your balance—whether you are active or not. Balance relies on your eyes, ears, muscles, and joints all working together with the brain. Your brain uses the information it receives to keep you upright. Now, if one of the body parts is a bit faulty, the brain is working with incorrect information, and you begin to lose balance. But all is not lost. We can teach the brain to react correctly by exercising the part that is a bit problematic.

The next problem is falls. If your brain isn't keeping you upright, you could easily fall. Falls are dangerous for seniors. Your bone density is not what it was 20 years ago. Your brittle bones may break during a fall, which will probably involve an operation and maybe weeks of inactivity while you heal. The statistics are not in your favor, too many elderly people die because of a fall.

If you fall, there is a high probability that you won't be able to get up, particularly if you are unfit. The important muscle groups to help you get up are your abs and your thighs. If either of these muscle groups are weak you will need help getting up. But what if there is no one around? One lady I know fell in her bathroom and she couldn't get up. She stayed in an apartment but wasn't acquainted with her neighbors. She lay helpless in the bathroom for three days, with nothing to eat and nothing to drink because she couldn't reach the taps. She tried banging on the pipes, but no one heard or took notice of the faint noise. A friend got worried when she didn't answer her phone. With the help of the landlord, they discovered her and called an ambulance. She had broken her femur. She went to the hospital, but the shock, the broken leg, and the dehydration led to her death.

I would like to address this issue with people who live alone. It is necessary to have an arrangement with a friend or relative that you will contact them every day by, let's say at 10 am. This is easy now that most people have cell phones and WhatsApp. If the friend doesn't hear from you, they must either get to your place as quickly as possible or use 911 to alert emergency personnel that something is wrong. We need to look after one another. If you are in another country, make sure you know the emergency number; you never know when you may need it.

So, get up and do the baseline test as described above. You don't have to do the test in order to start doing the exercise, but it does help you to see your improvement over time. It is a good idea to do the baseline test every month to spur you on to get better and better results.

Follow the suggested progress for the exercise. It may be necessary to spend a few more sessions on each step. Take note that it is a *suggested* progress. You may find that the first step is too easy after three sessions, then move on to the next step. If you find that a week is not enough, then make it two weeks or more. Only you can decide how you are handling each progressive step.

One thing I suggest is that you keep a journal of your progress. This can be done in a book or a file on the computer. My suggested format for this is below— you are welcome to change it as you see fit:

Date	Exercise	Reps	Comments
4/4/24	Single Leg Stance (Beginner)	5	I managed to do three repetitions with my eyes closed!

The next chapter will add another exercise to your selection of exercises. You will again need a stable chair to help you since the exercise deals with the shins. You will notice that we are spending quite a bit of time on the mid to lower body. Strength in those muscles will stabilize you and give you strength to get up when you fall.

CHAPTER 5
ESSENTIAL AND QUICK FITNESS ROUTINE #4: SHIN EXERCISES

Shin Exercises

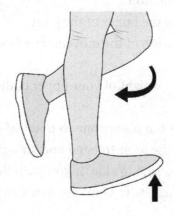

S o far, we have mainly concentrated on exercises that focus on our lower body, from the abs downwards. However, I have been very quiet about the most important and biggest joint in your body—your knee. It is almost a load-bearing joint. Your thigh bone (femur), shin bones (tibia & fibula), and kneecap (patella) make up the bones in this joint together with cartilage, muscle, nerves, tendons, and two menisci. The role of cartilage, muscles, and tendons is the same for the knee as it would be for anywhere else in the body.

This brings me to the meniscus—or plural menisci. The menisci lie between the femur and the tibia. One on the left side of the joint and one on the right. Its purpose is to:

- Be a shock absorber. Your knee joint receives punishment when you move around. When you are walking, there is minimal action for the menisci. Running, jumping, and any other intensive movement, bring out the true value of its shock absorber function.
- Prevent friction in the bones of the joint.
- Help the coordination of the movement when you walk, run, or dance.
- Support the entire weight of your upper body.

Your knees are robust but also prone to injury if you are not careful. Your knee allows the joint to bend and straighten, and there is a bit of leeway moving side to side. If you push the joint rapidly in a side motion, you may tear your meniscus, which will usually require an operation.

The exercise we will be discussing helps to strengthen the muscles of the knee and shin. We have dealt with abs, hips, and thighs. All of these are very important to help stabilize you during movement, but if we leave the knee and shin out of the mix, we will have a very vulnerable part of our body.

Your femur is the strongest bone in your body, while the tibia is the most vulnerable bone. Exercise strengthens the muscles surrounding the tibia, protecting it from breaking.

Just imagine breaking one of your shin bones—your tibia or fibula. Can you walk? Oh no, you cannot. The area will be painful and swollen. You will find it too painful to put any weight on, and the movement of your ankle and knee will be inhibited.

The leg will also be put in a plaster cast or a boot. You will be issued crutches for the first few weeks. It could take up to 12 weeks to heal. The crutches, a painful lower leg, and your cast will interfere with your normal daily activity. You will get used to the restriction, but it would be so much better if your shin muscles were stronger. Strong shin muscles will help protect your leg from being forced into weird positions which lead to breakage.

Now just think how much better life would be if your muscles were in tip-top condition to help you ward off injuries when falling. The muscles could even prevent the fall from taking place to start with.

WHY IS THIS ROUTINE ESSENTIAL?

If you live a sedentary life your feet and legs do not get the attention that they need. There are a few ways that you can give your feet, ankles, lower legs, and knees the exercise that will strengthen them and make them less likely to face broken bones. These exercises not only strengthen the necessary areas but will also help keep your balance. Most falls come from a lack of fitness and an inability to balance.

If you are a runner, or you play a sport that needs you to run—like soccer, tennis, baseball, or basketball—you may get shin splints. In this case, the sensible thing would be to prepare yourself by doing exercises that will strengthen your joints and muscles in your lower legs.

We often neglect our legs when we exercise. We seem to prefer to concentrate on the upper body and abs. A good workout works every facet of your body. I have already explained how strong thighs and abs can help prevent falls as well as how, with strong legs and abs, getting up from a fall is much easier. Of course, we want to avoid falls as much as possible, which is why a full-body workout will help.

Your Progress

You should do this exercise—regardless of which variation you choose—at least five times a week. The explanations will discuss the time you need for this exercise.

After one week:

You will become aware of how much your lower limb needs the exercise. Your ankles, calves, and shins will start to be more supple.

Shin splints are painful, but you should start to feel less pain during exercises or during walking or running.

After one month:

You will become aware that your lower limbs are functioning better and with less pain. The ankle and knee joints will be more supple, which means that there will be less pain. The discomfort that you probably felt before you started will disappear. You will find the exercise easier, no matter which variation you choose.

After three months:

- Your ankles will be stronger, and with this added strength, they will be more stable. This bodes well for preventing falls.
- Your walking style will improve due to the general increase of strength in the lower limbs. Your lower limbs will work with the upper limbs to give you a safe, energetic gait.
- Your lower limbs will get stronger, making them more compatible with your upper limbs. Each part of your lower body will work together with similar strength levels.
- Your shin splints will be healed, and your shins will be protected against developing them again.
- Your balance will improve as your lower body strength improves.

STEP-BY-STEP GUIDE THROUGH THE SHIN EXERCISE

Equipment: A chair. Preferably with no arms and wheels.

Instruction:

1. Sit on the chair with both feet flat on the floor.
2. Sit with your knees together and let your legs form a 90° angle.
3. Slowly raise your toes as high as they can go.
4. Hold for the count of five.
5. Rest for the count of three.
6. Repeat five times.

Difficulty Levels

Beginner: The exercise outlined above is the beginner's exercise.

Intermediate:

Equipment: A wall and you might like to have a friend or helper for support if needed the first few times you do this exercise.

Instruction:

1. Use the wall as support.
2. Stand about a foot away from the wall with your feet together.
3. Carefully lean back so that your head, shoulders, and hips are in contact with the wall. For this part you may feel more confident if your friend or helper is close by.
4. Raise your toes as far as you can.
5. Lower your toes until they are about an inch off the floor.
6. Raise your toes again.
7. Repeat this action 15 times.
8. Briefly rest before repeating the exercise twice more.

Advanced:

Equipment: Your chair.

Instruction:

1. Stand behind your chair.
2. Hold on to the back of your chair with your feet slightly apart. The distance between you and your chair must be such that your arms are extended but not stretched straight.
3. Flex your knees.

4. Extend your right leg as far back as it can go but keep your foot flat on the floor—keep your heel down.
5. Bend your left knee to accommodate the stretch.
6. Hold for 30 seconds—if you can't manage 30 seconds, you can build up to it.
7. Bring your right leg forward so that your right foot is next to your left foot.
8. Repeat with the left leg.

Expert:

Equipment: You need a staircase—or a plastic step like a child will use to reach a counter or the toilet. The handrail is there if you need some assistance, or you could also use your helper if you are feeling a bit wobbly.

Instruction:

1. Stand on the bottom step of a flight of stairs facing upwards—or stand on the plastic step.
2. Swing your right foot back to place the right heel on the floor with your toes facing upwards.
3. Bring your foot back to stand on the step.
4. Repeat this 15 times.
5. Change feet so the left foot swings back.

BEST PRACTICES

Some tips to help you on your way.

- I have not included any equipment other than the chair. So, to reiterate how to choose the chair:
- It must be a stable chair as you will depend on it to help your stability in some of the exercises.

- The chair shouldn't have arms because they will get in your way.
- It shouldn't have wheels.
- So, can you use a walker instead? Yes, you can but make sure that the Brake is engaged.
- Before you start your exercise session remember to warm up. At the end of the session, you need to cool down. My favorite cool-down is to gently stretch all your muscle groups before lying down with hands to your sides— similar to the corpse pose in Yoga. Settle your breathing and lie still for five minutes.

BALANCED LIVING: HOW TO INCORPORATE THIS EXERCISE INTO DAILY LIFE

When you commit to an exercise plan decide if you prefer to isolate a block of time in your diary or to snatch a few minutes here and there in your day. If you isolate a block of time, make sure not to answer the phone or door for the whole session. Play some relaxing music and devote the time to yourself for your exercises.

If you prefer to snatch a few minutes at a time here are a few suggestions to help you do so consistently:

- Whenever you are standing somewhere waiting, do two or three exercises. You could be waiting for a store to open, in line at a store, or waiting for the kettle to boil. We all have those wasted minutes in a day.
- Watching your favorite program: You could actually do your entire routine while watching. If you are watching something that needs a bit more concentration, keep your exercise time for the commercial breaks. As every program

on TV needs funding, there will be quite a few ad breaks where you can do one or two of your exercises per break. Let's presume that there are four ad breaks, each lasting two minutes, you have saved about eight minutes for exercising.

- If you are having a three-course meal at home, do about 5 minutes of exercise before starting. Take another five-minute exercise break while waiting for the main course. There is usually quite a long break after the main course to "make room for" dessert. You could easily rack up 15 to 20 minutes during the meal.
- If you are talking to a friend on the phone, try to get a few reps of your favorite exercise.
- Exercise for 10 minutes before a meal.
- Do a couple of reps before bed. Include a warm-down routine before you climb into bed to help you relax.

For the next few suggestions, just a word of warning for anyone who has a health condition: Ignore these suggestions or only do them if you are sure that it is safe to do so. Make sure to talk to your healthcare practitioner before starting any form of exercise.

- When going shopping park your car as far away from the entrance as possible.
- Use stairs instead of the elevator or the escalator.
- Do not use the moving walkway at an airport.
- If you are traveling by bus, get off one stop before—or after—your stop.

If you are still working, there are many exercises that you can do at your desk.

SEGUE

There is hardly a chronic condition that can't be helped by getting
more active. As you get fitter you will notice an improvement in
your chronic conditions. You will find that you sleep better, and
you have more energy. Some other conditions that are generally
improved with an active lifestyle include:

- improved heart conditions
- lowering your blood pressure
- controlling weight
- improved muscle tone
- becoming positive about life in general.
- impro general. Centration and brain function
- a generally healthier and happier life

By now you have done exercises that impact muscle groups from
the abs down to your feet. These exercises are very important for
helping you stay balanced in all the meanings of the word. As you
get older your balance declines due to inactivity or damage. Bad
balance invites falls. For seniors, falls can be dangerous and sometimes lead to death. A broken bone needs surgery and surgery can
have dangerous complications. If they survive the surgery, some
weeks of inactivity follow as your break mends. An inactive senior
is a disaster waiting to happen. A dance teacher that I know broke
her hip in a fall. Because she was extremely fit, she was soon on
her feet, holding onto her hospital bed while she did plies and
rises. The doctors were amazed at how quickly she recovered. The
stronger your lower body is the quicker you will recover from a
fall.

Exercise Program

Your exercise program can include all the exercises discussed so far or you can select those exercises that you feel your body needs. While it is best to exercise for at least 30 minutes per day, there is no law that says it must be 30 continuous minutes. You could do 10 minutes when you get up, then 10 minutes at some stage during the day, and your last 10 minutes can be before your evening meal. The only problem with breaking it up this way is that you will need to warm up and cool down three times a day rather than just once.

Some days a 30-minute session will not be possible. Then you will need to grab whatever opportunities come up on that day.

Warm-Up

There are several ways you can warm up for your exercise session. My favorites are:

- Breathing. I like rectangular breathing but there are many other types of breathing that you can try. With rectangular breathing, you imagine a rectangle like a door or a window. Your inhale comes on the short side and the exhale on the long side. I like to breathe in for the count of four (climbing up the short side of your rectangle) and breathe out for ten (going along the long side). The reason I like this breathing exercise—which was a favorite in treating COVID-19—is that you have to control your exhale; otherwise, you will find it hard to reach the count of 10. You can try other counts until you find the right rhythm for you. Just remember that there must be a distinct difference in the counts for the inhale and the exhale.

- Stretching. Start at the top of your body. Stretch the neck muscles then the shoulders, arms, lower back, all the way down to your toes.

Cool-Down

Incorporate yoga poses in your cool-down—I like to do the corpse pose here. Lie down, preferably on your bed because you might get stuck if you lie on the floor. Now, just as you stretch every part of your body in the warm-up, you are going to consciously relax every muscle, starting with your toes and working up to the neck. Continue to lie down as you do a breathing exercise. When you feel relaxed, slowly get up. Just be careful as you get up because you may experience slight dizziness.

In the next chapter, we are going to continue with the lower leg as we explore calf raises.

Be Part of the Balance Revolution!

"Aging is not lost youth but a new stage of opportunity and strength."

BETTY FRIEDAN

Many of us see the value in improving our balance as we get older. Perhaps a fall scares us, or maybe we just feel a little less steady on our feet than we used to. It makes us aware of one of the most frightening aspects of aging. We've all heard of older people who rarely leave their homes because of the risk of falling or the difficulty they have with moving around, and we don't want that to be us.

The problem for many people is, they get that far, and they don't know what to do about it. They need not only clear guidance to help them improve their balance but also the confidence that if they commit to it, they really can make a difference to their quality of life going forward.

By this stage in the book, you've seen how easily these exercises can be integrated into your life – no matter how busy you are. So it's at this stage in our journey together that I'd like to ask you to take a moment to help all those people who have concerns about their balance but don't have a clue what to do about it.

"But what can I do?" you're thinking, and the answer is surprisingly simple. By doing nothing more than taking a couple of minutes to leave a review, you'll make this book more visible to the people who are looking for it.

By leaving a review of this book on Amazon, you'll help anyone who's searching for ways to improve their balance find the information that will help them.

Countless people need this guidance, and balance is so important in later life that I'm determined to help them find it. With your help, I'll be able to reach many more people – and that means improved quality of life all over the country.

Thank you so much for your support. We can make so much difference when we work together.

Scan the QR code to leave a review:

CHAPTER 6
ESSENTIAL AND QUICK FITNESS ROUTINE #5: CALF RAISES

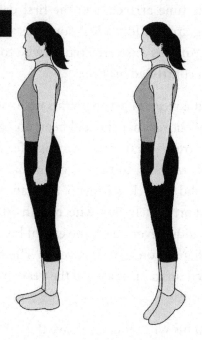

Calf Raises

W hen Wally was in college, he joined the track team. He was quite good in short races, but he excelled in cross-country. He was as fit as a fiddle.

When he got his first job after college, he tried to keep up with his running, but he found that as an intern at a law firm, he always brought mounds of work home. When he was single, he found little time for his running, and once he got married and when the children came, his running time became almost non-existent. It was a short stretch to drop it completely. He was always promising that he would have more time to resume his running "next year." Then suddenly, as happens in life, "next year" was the year he planned to retire and would definitely have more time.

And so, the time arrived, and the first day of his retirement saw him pacing around like a lost soul. His wife suggested that he go for a run. And his answer? "Yep, maybe tomorrow." So, procrastination still controlled his time.

After about a week of getting in his wife's way as she went through the normal chores that she had been doing for many years, he got up with a fresh perspective on his life. He entered the kitchen wearing his trainers, to the delight of his wife. He grabbed a light breakfast, did a quick warm-up, and ran down the garden path to the road. Fortunately, his wife had insisted that he take his cell phone. He didn't even reach the end of his block when the pain hit, and he collapsed on the grass verge. The pain started in his ankle and traveled up to his knee. All the years of not training came back to roost.

He phoned his wife, and she drove the car to pick him up and take him to the doctor.

Fortunately, there were no breaks, but a break would heal quicker than a torn ligament. His doctor berated him gently for trying to pick up where he had left off so many years before. He needed to give his leg time to heal so he was banned from doing any exercise that would make the tear worse.

"Six weeks," declared the doctor, " then I need to see you again before I allow you to run again."

At the end of six weeks, he went back to the doctor. The doctor explained what had happened and why it had happened.

"After so many sedentary years, your muscles and tendons had shrunk. There was no way you could pick up running again without a plan to get fit first. Your ankle, calf, and knee need stretching. I want you to do calf raises for three weeks. Then come and see me again, and we can introduce more exercises to make your leg joints and muscles strong enough to start running again. And don't forget to warm up before you start."

The doctor gave Wally a pamphlet with some good warm-up exercises and calf raises. Wally followed the doctor's instructions and could feel the improvement daily. His ankles felt more stable, and walking became easier. He felt more energetic and the strength in his legs was getting better and better.

WHY THIS EXERCISE?

Calf Raises have many benefits. Your calves will become stronger and with their strength comes better balance. The exercise targets the two muscles behind your shin, helps extend your hamstrings, and reduces stress on the Achilles tendon. You will find that you are comfortable walking on any surface, whether it is smooth, flat, stony, and rough. Other benefits include:

- As your calves get stronger, so do your ankles and your feet and the strength helps your stability.
- Many of the exercises in the previous chapters helped you exercise your lower body. Introducing calf raises strengthens all the muscles in your lower body.
- If you wish to become a competitive runner, calf raises help. Your strides become longer as your confidence builds —all due to stronger calf muscles. Longer strides mean that you will shave some time off your best race.
- The more toned your calf muscles become, the less your chance of injury.
- Calf raises also save your joints from injury. If you do a lot of running, strong calves will help your feet hit the tarmac softly thus preventing jars on your joints.
- There is an increase in blood flow which means the heart does not have to work extra hard to ensure that the blood can flow easily throughout your body.

Expected Progress

Doing this exercise five times a week will have a marked improvement in your gait. Your feet will connect with the floor softly but strongly.

After one week:

- You will have gained more strength in your lower body, particularly in your calves.
- You will notice a slight change in the appearance of your calves.

After one month:

- Your ankles will be stronger, and your stance will be firmer.
- Your calves will be stronger and will also be toned in appearance.

After three months:

- You will have more confidence in walking and running as you will feel more stable. Before you might have been a bit unsteady while walking, or you might have hesitated when you came to a curb, but now you will walk much more confidently.
- Your ankles will be stronger, and you will be able to rotate them more easily. A shuffling walk could also have been caused by worrying about your weak ankles.
- Your posture will be much better now that you don't have to bend over to make sure that your feet and ankles behave. Better posture places less strain on your legs and your back.

HOW TO PROPERLY DO CALF RAISES: STEP-BY-STEP GUIDE

Equipment: Your trusty chair. Make sure that you can sit comfortably with your feet flat on the floor.

Instructions:

1. This is a seated exercise. Sit with a straight back and with your feet about a hip-width apart, flat on the floor.

2. Adjust your feet backwards so that your heels are behind your knees but your feet are still flat on the floor.
3. Rise up onto your toes as high as possible.
4. Hold for the count of 10 then gently lower your heels until your feet are flat on the floor.
5. Repeat 10 times.

Difficulty Levels

Beginner: The exercise as described above is the beginner exercise

Intermediate:

- Stand behind the back of the chair with your feet slightly apart. Hold onto the chair for this variant.
- Make sure you are standing tall and that you do not compromise your posture as you go through the exercise.
- Exercise each leg separately. Rise up onto the toes of your right foot and hold for the count of 10.
- Gently lower your foot and repeat with the left foot.
- Rest, then repeat the entire exercise five times.

Advanced:

- Stand behind the chair, holding onto the back.
- Stand with your feet flat on the ground, slightly apart. Make sure you are standing tall and that you do not compromise your posture as you go through the exercise.
- Rise up as high as you can on both feet. Hold for the count of 10.
- Gently lower your feet.
- Repeat at least five times.

Expert: This is essentially the same as the advanced exercise, but you will hold the pose for the count of 20 and you will do at least 10 repetitions.

Best Practices

Some tips to help you get the best results.

- When doing the exercise, put your heart and soul into the effort, but don't rush it. The slower you do it, the more strength you build.
- Try to get a good rhythm as you go. Playing music can help.
- Watch your posture. Keep your back straight and your chest tall.
- If you are not getting the best results, the number of repetitions may be too low. It is fine to increase the number of reps, but try to keep the count between 10 and 30.

BALANCED LIVING: HOW TO INCORPORATE THIS EXERCISE INTO DAILY LIFE

We all—even pensioners—are so busy nowadays that we often battle to find the time to exercise. Or are we just trying to find an excuse that may be acceptable? If you are always making excuses, try to figure out why. It may be that the form of exercise that you are choosing is not for you. Your exercise time should be enjoyable. If you enjoy this form of exercise, you will make time if necessary.

The best thing is to write in your journal for half an hour every day. Once you have written it down, you are more likely to keep the engagement with yourself.

Remember that you are doing this for yourself, not for a partner, a friend, or a family member. This is for you. For your fitness so that you can have a healthy life.

While it is best to exercise in a set half hour, we need to acknowledge that a bit of exercise is better than no exercise. So, if you honestly can only find 10 minutes then use that 10 minute. You may be able to find two more-time frames that will help you get your 30 minutes of exercise for the day.

It always helps if you plan your exercise time and write it down. Our minds are funny things. If we have consciously allocated time to something, we will keep to the plan. But if you decide to see what the day brings and then allocate time, it is all too easy to evade the session. We have discussed making use of spare time earlier in the book, but I will reiterate it here again.

- Calf raisers can be done while waiting in a line or waiting for the kettle to boil. I can hear you already starting to object! "But then everyone will see it and will laugh at me." Most people you won't see again, so what does it matter? And if you do see them, tell them that you are preparing for a fit retirement.
- When reaching for an item high up, it is ideal to do a few calf raises before grabbing it.
- While the elevator is traveling to your floor, get a few calf raises in there.
- When you go shopping, do a calf raise when reaching for an item on the shelf. Do a few more when you are waiting

in line. When you are unpacking your items at the till, try to get a couple of calf raises in. When you get home do a calf raiser for every item you pack away.

A Habit

Doing exercises should become a habit. There are many theories on what it means to develop a habit. Some authorities say that you need to do the desired action nine times for it to become a habit. Others say you need to do it 90 times before it becomes a habit. And then there is a school of thought that it takes 21 days to formulate a habit (Clear, 2018).

I have found that doing something for 21 days does establish it as a habit. So, if you do the planned exercise routine for 21 days, it will, more than likely, become a habit.

Forming an exercise habit is important if you want to make your senior years productive. Seniors who keep fit get a lot more enjoyment out of life than those who do not. Once you have retired it is too easy to sink into being a couch potato. You really must make a conscious decision to be active.

SEGUE

You are starting to get quite a few exercises in your armory, and if you have been getting your 30 minutes per day, you should be feeling much better than when you started.

Did you identify with Wally at all? It is very easy to procrastinate. We can always find time to play games on our cell phones so why is it so hard to find the time to exercise? I am not saying don't play games on your phone, I am saying prioritize your exercise time.

Cell phone games can be mindless, or they can be mindful. There are games like Wordle (a word game) and Nerdle (a math game) that are marvelous for keeping our senior brains sharp. So, if you must play games, play games that exercise your brain, it will help stave off dementia.

When you decide to start an exercise program, one way to keep your brain engaged is by paying a bit of attention to your clothing. First, make sure to choose comfortable, loose-fitting clothing. Then, select a couple of outfits so that your brain will start to associate the clothing with the exercise time. For example, if you are going to walk, put on the same pair of trainers each time you set out. When you are doing the exercises in this book always do it in similar clothing and in the same place. This will help build up the exercise habit. You are going to have to be stern with yourself in the early days of generating a habit, but it does get easier as you go.

Recording your progress will also help you stay on the exercise course. You could select a day—I do Friday—and make notes of how many reps you were able to do. Then, compare it to the previous week or weeks and see how you have improved.

I also find it useful to set a target—don't make it too easy—and to reward yourself when you reach that target. The reward shouldn't be edible like that donut that is sitting in your fridge. Maybe you could buy a magazine that you have always left on the shelf because it was expensive. You could also buy a new outfit. I like to pop a small amount of money into a jar—like people do with swear jars—and when there is enough money in there, I will buy a treat.

In the next chapter, we will tackle toe-to-heel walking. This is a very important exercise for helping you keep your balance. Doctors often use it to assess your ability to balance.

Another exercise that doctors use to test your balance is to ask you to walk with your eyes closed. By the end of this book, you will pass all balance tests with flying colors.

CHAPTER 7
ESSENTIAL AND QUICK FITNESS ROUTINE #6: HEEL TO TOE WALK

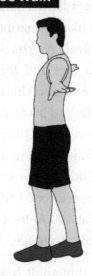

Heel to Toe Walk

All the exercises we have discussed and included in our exercise routine have been selected to fight the balance war that occurs as we age. While your body may let you down, your brain can be trained to take over. As you practice the exercises, the brain says, "Ah, yes. I know those moves, so I need to make sure that my body stays upright and doesn't fall."

When you reach 60, you need to incorporate balance exercises into your exercise regimen—if you haven't already started. The more balanced you are, the less likely you are to fall, and as we have mentioned, falls can be lethal. They can lead to broken bones or even death. Broken bones mend easily when you are young, but with age, mending becomes difficult, and bones take longer to heal.

As you grow older, it gets harder and harder to maneuver your body. Even trivial things like navigating through uneven sidewalks can be a frustrating ordeal. As you age your general flexibility deteriorates. When your legs and feet lose their flexibility, you start finding it so much easier to shuffle as you walk. While shuffling will get you from place to place, it adds years to your life. You will look much older than you actually are. The next thing to go will be your posture. While there is nothing wrong with looking your age, you certainly don't want to look older. The straighter your posture, the more coordinated your walking style will be and the better you will feel about yourself. Especially when it makes people gasp when they hear your age.

It's not all about vanity, though. It is about feeling and moving as well as you can, about having a good quality of life. You need to start believing that your age does not define you, that age is just a number.

Get started on this exercise as soon as you can. A heel-to-toe Walk will stretch your entire foot, including the ankles, making the foot more flexible. More flexible feet will make walking easier, and you will look good while walking. You will also be able to walk further and be quicker.

ANATOMY OF WALKING

Our normal mode of walking on a reasonable surface is as follows:

1. We bend the knee as the toes leave the ground.
2. We set the heel down.
3. We roll through the foot to the ball of our foot.
4. As our toes leave the ground, we are back to the first point.

When walking upstairs or downstairs we will usually let our toes strike first.

If the surface is uneven and full of stones, we walk much more carefully. It might be easier to let our toes strike first.

Heel Striking

This style is a normal walking style, but if you are using it as an exercise, all the action must be deliberate and thoughtful. You let your heel strike the floor first and then smoothly roll through the foot to the ball of the foot. As the roll of the foot reaches the toes the other leg is getting ready to move. The roll onto the toes gives added impetus to the other leg.

Toe Striking

This style of walking can look a bit awkward, but we use it when walking or running on the spot. We also use it when we are climbing stairs. Runners will often prefer this method to the heel-striking method. As with heel-striking, the action of the foot is a rolling action. The toes hit the ground first and then roll through the ball of the foot to the heel. Sometimes in running, the heel does not touch the ground. If you want to get a good understanding of this style walk backward—there is no way that your heel can touch first if you are walking backward.

Posture While Walking

Starting from the feet upwards:

- Feet: Should always point forwards.
- Knees: The back knee should be flexed. Keep it bent as it passes the standing foot. Your weight shifts as your knee goes forward.
- Engage your glutes as you walk.
- This one might feel a bit strange: Your thumbs should always be pointing forward. This helps keep your shoulders upright.
- Engage your core.
- Keep your shoulders upright.
- Keep your chin parallel to the ground.

BENEFITS OF HEEL-TO-TOE WALKING

This exercise has several benefits:

- It builds stability while we are standing or walking. We know that we become less stable as we age, so any exercise that enhances stability has to be included in our bank of exercises.
- It helps keep our balance while we walk up or down stairs.
- It adds strength to our legs which helps us stand up from a seated position.
- We tackle jobs around the house more readily when we don't have to worry about losing balance.
- Walking becomes easier and less energy-intensive so we can extend our usual walking distance.
- It helps with coordinating our movements around the house.

So how do you achieve these benefits? By practicing daily. You should see the following benefits:

After one week:

- You should see an improvement in your coordination.
- You will experience better focus.
- Your ankles will be stronger.

After one month:

- Your balance will improve.
- Your whole leg will be stronger.
- Your gait and posture will improve.

After three months:

- Your balance and stability will be much improved.
- Your posture will have improved.
- You will look good as your gait has improved.

INSTRUCTIONS FOR HEEL-TO-TOE WALKING

General Instructions

This exercise is difficult to do to begin with, but as you get better at it, you will see a marked improvement in your balance. Your balance will be challenged at the start, so we need to take some precautions.

Make sure you have a wall or counter next to you so that you can grab onto it if you tend to lose your balance. A passage or corridor is the ideal place to do this exercise.

If you use a walker, you can do this exercise while holding onto it. Every day try to do at least four steps without the walker. I suggest you try that towards the end of your exercise.

Try to select a smooth surface to do this exercise. If you do it on a rough path first, you need a handrail or other form of support. Secondly, the rough terrain will easily cause you to lose your balance. So, it's preferable to do this exercise inside. Make sure there are no loose carpets on your course.

The Exercise (Step-By-Step)

1. Hold onto the wall, counter, or walker. Put your dominant foot in front of your other foot so that the heel of the dominant foot touches the toes of the other foot.

2. Bring your other foot in front of the dominant foot, heel to toe. Leave the wall if you feel confident.

3. Watch your posture: Keep your chin parallel to the ground. I kept my shoulders relaxed, eyes open and continued with the heel-to-toe motion.

4. When you reach the end of your passage turn and repeat.

5. Stabilize yourself before continuing with your heel-to-toe walk.

Difficulty Levels:

Beginner: As is explained above. Try to do at least 30 steps.

Intermediate:

- Do the same as before but add a twist to it: Engage your brain in a task while you are doing the exercise. This tests the ability of the brain to multitask.
- A simple brain task could be naming things like names, products, or towns beginning with letters of the alphabet and going from A to Z. For example, if you chose a boy's name, you could cite Adam, Barry, Chad, etc.
- This task splits the attention and concentration between the task and your walking.

Advanced:

- The exercise is the same as for beginners, but you will not be using any aids to help your balance, so there will be no wall, and your walker has been retired.
- Do an exaggerated roll of the foot before placing it. Place your heel while your toes face upwards. Roll through the foot until your toes touch the ground. Place the other foot on the heel and slowly roll through the foot until the toes

are placed. You may still like to have a wall or counter close by.

Expert: This is the same as the previous stage but speed up your walking. You might like to have a friend close by in case you lose balance.

MECHANICS OF HEEL-TO-TOE WALKING

As with any exercise program, the idea is to start slowly, particularly if you are not very fit. This exercise works on all your lower body muscle groups, including the abs. It is one of a few exercises that will tone and strengthen your ankles. Strengthening the ankles will help your stability and lessen your propensity to fall.

Have you ever considered that your feet are the body's shock absorbers? They cushion your full body weight as you walk. Stability starts in your feet, which is why it is important to do strengthening exercises.

Your footwear must be comfortable particularly when exercising or walking. High heels will make you unstable in old age even if you have worn high heels all your adult life. When buying new shoes make sure that they have low heels, give good support, and have a non-slip sole.

When you start exercising, and this includes all standing exercises, make sure that there is something that you can grab onto if you get a bit wobbly. This can be the wall, a counter, a chair, or even a friend.

Another aspect of maintaining your balance is watching your posture. Stand as straight as you can and relax your shoulders. Your chin should be kept parallel to the ground. If you allow your shoulders to stoop, you will be offsetting your weight, as your shoulders and upper body will be inclining forward. Keep your eyes focused straight ahead.

BALANCED LIVING

How to Incorporate This Exercise into Daily Life

Sometimes, we find it hard to find time to exercise. If we can find a way to do them as we go about our chores, it will take away some of the guilt we may feel. This exercise is particularly easy to incorporate into our daily lives.

• As you walk from one room to another, you can do the heel-to-toe walk. You probably walk to various rooms at least ten times a day. You walk to the kitchen to get your meals and something to drink. You go to the bathroom at least three times a day. So those two rooms alone can clock up ten different occasions you walked around your home.

• When you are doing chores around the house, you can incorporate heel-to-toe walking.

• If you have a choice between an elevator or the stairs, take the stairs. If you are confident about your grasp of the heel-to-toe movement and you have reached the advanced or expert status you could try the heel-to-toe movement as you walk up and down the stairs.

• If you have access to a treadmill, you can get a few heel-to-toe reps under your belt.

- At the supermarket:

  - Try using the heel-to-toe walk when you walk down the aisles.
  - Use this style of walking to get from your car to the supermarket.
  - It can also be done as you unpack your shopping or at any time you walk from your car to your house or shop.

- If you practice rolling through your foot while you are watching TV, the movement is not quite as effective, but your ankles will get a workout. Sit with your legs slightly extended in front of you. You can do both feet together or one at a time. I will explain using both feet:

  - Lift your toes off the ground as far as you can so that only your heels are in contact with the floor.
  - Lower your toes in a rolling motion until your foot is flat on the floor, then raise your heels as high as you can.
  - The closer your legs are to forming a 90° angle with your thighs, the higher you will get onto your toes.

- At the end of the day try a few minutes of heel-to-toe walking as a cool-down in preparation for bed.

SEGUE

If you haven't exercised for a while this is a nice, light exercise to do. It might be fairly easy and not need too much in the line of stamina, but it is a powerful exercise to help your mind and body stay balanced.

Your posture is extremely important when you are walking. Your head, neck, and spine should be in a straight line. Get someone to put a walking stick from your head down your back. Adjust your posture until the walking stick lies close to your head and back. Drop your shoulders but keep them relaxed and tighten your abs.

This exercise works the toes, the feet, the ankle, the entire leg, and the abs—as long as you keep a good posture. It is one of the few exercises that work the ankles. A supple ankle helps keep you balanced. When you lose that balance, you could fall, and as we have already discussed, falling is dangerous but, unfortunately, quite common.

When you exercise, pay attention to your clothing and your shoes. Clothing should be loose so that it doesn't restrict your movement. You can exercise with bare feet or with shoes. Bare feet are fine if you are used to walking barefoot. Shoes should be light and flexible so that they don't restrict your movement. You can get proper exercise socks that have cleats on the soles—not cleats like football boots; the cleats on the socks are rubbery.

When you go for a walk, pay close attention to how you use your feet. We don't want a shuffle since it is the type of movement that ages you fast. Concentrate on your heel, hitting the ground first, then roll through the foot until your toes peel off the ground to take the next step. Make sure that the surface is smooth, as a rough surface can be very difficult to walk on.

Before starting any exercise routine, you must do a warm-up. The warm-up can be as simple as walking on the spot, going for a five-minute walk, or a short jog. After the session cool down.

Remember that if you are fit, you will be healthier, have more energy, sleep better, and stay positive more easily, no matter what life flings at you.

In the next chapter, we are going to look at marching in place.

CHAPTER 8
ESSENTIAL AND QUICK FITNESS ROUTINE #7: MARCHING IN PLACE

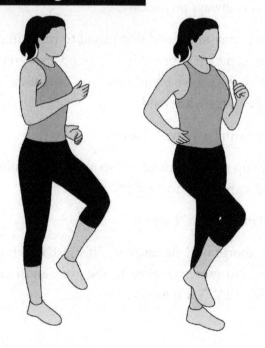

Marching in Place

I grabbed my gym bag while smothering a deep sigh. The car was in for a service, and if I was really serious about getting fit and losing weight, I needed to either get an Uber—a bit more than I could afford—or walk two blocks to catch the bus that would drop me two blocks away from the gym. If I am walking four blocks to get to the gym, isn't that a good reason to skip the gym? Why walk those four blocks if I am not going to go to the gym? And I realized I would have to walk those four blocks to get home. What to do? Oh, I wish there was a magic carpet to get me to the gym. Or I wish I could get fit just by staying at home! How about getting fit, sitting on the couch, eating ice cream, and watching Netflix?

As I verbalized that last thought, I realized how childish I was being. I was grown up, and I did need to get fit; my kids and grandkids were always on my case.

I decided to phone my friend that I used to run with, Garland. He always cheered me up. A breathless Garland answered the phone. I asked her why she was so breathless. "You caught me in the middle of my home exercises," she said.

"You are exercising at home?" I asked.

"Yeah. I gave up my gym membership about two months ago when I discovered a great way to keep fit."

Tell me, tell me, tell me," I asked.

"Keep your shorts on " he laughed. "It's just walking, walking in place that is! No more traveling to the gym, and I can even do it while watching TV. Try it tomorrow.

As I said goodbye and put the phone down, a frisson of excitement traveled down my body to stop as butterflies in my tummy. I couldn't wait until the next day. I hoped it would do as much for me as it does for him, or I would never hear the end of it.

SOLUTIONS TO PHYSICAL PROBLEMS

There are many advantages to doing the Marching in Place routine. There is definitely a fitness benefit, but you will be amazed at how much better your balance issues are. All it requires is for you to do this routine every day, especially at the start.

Fit people can fight germs much more effectively. This means that they will have fewer sick days, as their system is geared to fighting infections.

Seniors often suffer from balance problems. This exercise will help you adjust more quickly to changes in posture. One way people lose balance is by quickly changing direction, which can lead to dizziness and an inability to remain standing.

As you get older, you often worry about moving around because of the risks of falling. Inactive seniors become weaker and, therefore, battle to fight off colds, flu, and other more serious infections. However, you don't need to worry since this walking-in-place exercise is the answer you need to various health issues.

WHY IS THIS ROUTINE ESSENTIAL?

Walking is one of the most natural movements that we do. We start as children, and barring accidents or ill health, we continue to do it until the end. We know that we need to keep active in order to live a satisfying life. What easier activity is there? Well, yes, walking—or marching—on the spot is just as good as going for an outside walk or hike. The beauty of it is that you don't need to spend vast amounts of money, and you don't need a gym. You can get some exercise just by walking around your home doing chores.

Walking, whether around the house, on the spot, or taking a hike outside, burns calories and makes your feet, ankles, legs, and knees supple. Walking on the spot has the following benefits:

- It is low impact. Running is high impact, which is why so many professionals or competitors end up having knee problems. Walking does not have the same impact on your muscles, yet it exercises all your mid to lower muscles, like your abs, glutes, and legs, including the knees, ankles, and feet.
- It is free of charge. Now, everyone likes a bargain, so this fact makes walking on the spot a very attractive form of exercise. In today's world, gas is expensive, and you are going to have to rely on some form of gas-reliant vehicle to get you to the gym. So, I could also advocate that staying at home to exercise is one up for conservation! Your bank account will also be smiling!
- You can do this exercise anywhere. If you go on holiday, there is no bulky equipment to pack. If you go to the beach, you can practice it there. I know that most of us are a bit self-conscious, so walking on the spot in public may deter you. Come on! You have reached a time in your life when you can do anything, and people accept that old people sometimes do weird things.
- If you are watching your diet and you need to burn some calories, while it won't burn as much as running or working out in a gym, it does burn calories. The whole idea is to exercise to raise your heart rate. You may get

some scoffers who don't understand that you are getting enough exercise without bench presses and so on.

- This exercise does not need equipment, but if you have access to a treadmill, give walking on the spot a try. Start on a low setting and increase it as you get better and fitter.
- Walking on the spot is perfect exercise for seniors suffering from osteoporosis or knee damage. It is gentle so your bones and any inflamed body parts will not be injured.
- If you have high blood pressure or any other cardiac problem, walking on the spot is a safe form of exercise. It can reduce your blood pressure and be beneficial to your heart.
- If you do the exercise for 30 minutes per day, you will find an improvement in your legs and joints. I know that 30 minutes sounds like a lot but put on your favorite CD or log in to Spotify and enjoy the music as you walk. Some days you may not be able to isolate 30 minutes due to appointments, visitors, or other distractions. Well, on those days, try to get 30 minutes in via 10 minutes or 15 minutes here and there in the day. It is not as beneficial as a 30-minute session, but it is better than not doing it at all. Remember, the idea behind exercise is to raise your heart rate, and 30 minutes will do that adequately, which means you may not get the same result if you break that 30 minutes up into smaller sessions.
- If you get bored during your 30-minute stint, listen to music, turn on the TV and watch your favorite show, or listen to a podcast—this last suggestion also gives your brain a bit of a workout.
- You can get more out of your session if you engage your arms as well. Tuck your elbows into your waist and start using them as you walk on the spot. When you walk

normally you don't even think of your arm movements, so we want the same arm movements here—swing those arms to get a full-body workout.

- If you normally have a walking aid—like a walking stick or a walker—you can use it while you are walking on the spot. Eventually, you will have enough confidence to walk without it, but stay close to a chair, wall, or counter in case you feel a bit insecure.

PREPARING FOR YOUR 30-MINUTE SESSION

If you want your brain and body to take these sessions seriously, you need to dress the part and prepare your muscles:

- Wear loose clothing. Tight pants such as jeans will restrict your movements.
- Get a good pair of walking shoes. These will support your feet correctly.
- Do a quick warm-up like stretches or lunges.

What to Expect

As you go through the exercise every day, you will likely see or experience some good changes.

After one week:

- Your circulation will improve—even if you can't feel it, your doctor will be able to pick it up.
- The muscles in your lower limbs will feel more toned.
- You may be surprised by the increase in your energy levels.

After one month:

- Your balance and stability will be much better.
- You will find that the muscles in your lower limbs, like your calves, are more defined.

After three months:

- The muscles in your lower limbs will be stronger and more defined.
- Your heart function and your blood pressure will show an improvement.
- Your gait while walking casually will be improved.

HOW TO PROPERLY DO MARCHING IN PLACE

Step-by-Step Guide

Equipment: A chair, the wall, a counter, or a friend. You won't use them, but they'll be there in case you become unstable.

Goals: I have prepared a sample of how you can work and what you can expect to cover. This table is merely a suggestion, you can adjust it as you wish.

Week	Minutes per day	Number of days
1	10	4
2	15	5
3	15	5
4	20	6
5	20	6
6	30	5
7	30	5
8 onwards	30	5

Instructions:

1. Set boundaries so that you have a safety net in case you lose your balance. You can set a chair in front of you, stand near a wall, counter, or other furniture, or do the exercise near a friend who you can grab onto. You could also stand in a corner, so the wall is available on your right or left side.
2. Stand straight with your chin parallel to the ground. Tuck your elbows into your waist to start with your arms, forming a 90° angle. Keep your feet hip-width apart.
3. Your right arm works with your left leg, and your left arm works with your right leg—exactly as it would be if you were out taking a stroll.
4. Lift your right knee as high as is comfortable as you swing your left arm forward. The more you swing the arm, the more exercise it gets.
5. Lower the leg and bring the arm back to the starting position as you get ready to repeat with your left leg.

6. Repeat for the designated time.

Difficulty Levels

- **Beginner:** Exactly as it is described above.
- **Intermediate:** Try to march faster and lift the knee higher. You can also put a bit more of a punch into your arm movements.
- **Advanced:** The same as with the intermediate level but put in about four actual steps every five minutes. Your arms could do punching action.
- **Expert:** The same as for the advanced level, but when you put in some actual steps, alternate them sideways, forwards, and backward.

Additional information

When you are taking actual steps, make sure that your crutch—chair, wall, etc.—is always near enough to prevent you from falling.

Change the tempo of your movements so some steps will be fast and others slow. If you play music, you can choose different tempos. Make sure to keep your breathing regular.

AVOID THESE MISTAKES

Some of the mistakes mentioned deal more with walking or hiking than walking on the spot. I am aware that some of you will want to transfer from walking on the spot to using walking outside as your exercise for the day.

Your Walking Stride

When you go for a walk, make sure that your stride is comfortable. Don't try to match your stride to anyone else's. Taller people will have a longer stride than shorter people. If you try to make your stride too long, it will be uncomfortable, make your gait a bit comical, and hurt your shins and feet.

When you walk, make sure that your back leg pushes off the ground to propel you forward and that you roll through the standing foot so that the toes can push you forward.

Footwear

We have already discussed this a bit. However, if you wear ill-fitting shoes, you are setting yourself up for some health issues like Plantar fasciitis, knee issues, and sore leg muscles.

You need lightweight walking shoes that give your foot plenty of support. The sole must be thick enough to protect your feet on rough ground. The soles should also not be stiff, as that will place a strain on your entire foot. Thus, a good walking shoe needs to be a bit flexible.

Examine your shoes frequently to ensure that you replace them timeously. Badly worn shoes are bad for your feet and legs.

Your feet are liable to swell a bit while walking, so it might be an idea to get a shoe that is slightly bigger than you usually wear.

It is best if you buy your shoes from a specialist sports shop where you can be fitted with the correct shoe for you.

Walking Flat-Footed

Make sure that you roll through your feet as you walk. The heel should be the first part to hit the ground. Then, as the foot prepares for the next step, roll through the sole into the toes, which will then push you off into the next step.

Be wary if Your foot slaps onto the ground or if you do not roll through the standing foot. Both of these could lead to muscle damage to the leg.

Use Your Arms

Moving your arms while walking will counterbalance your foot-work. When you are just strolling, it is normal for your arms to swing a little, but when you are walking as exercise, you need to bend your arms and move them intentionally. This way, you exercise your upper body as well.

Look Where You Are Going

Do not walk with your head looking down. This will distort your posture and may also affect your balance. Good posture will help you walk faster and avoid accidents. Your chin should always be parallel to the ground.

General Posture

Posture is important when you are walking since it gives you a better appearance and prevents backache.

You may be tempted to walk leaning forward. While that might be acceptable for walking up a very steep incline, generally it is not good as you upset your balance, making you more inclined to fall.

The best posture has been described above—head up and chin parallel to the ground.

Keep Hydrated

Drink a glass of water a couple of hours before you exercise. Take some water with you, take frequent sips, and then have a big glass when you get home.

Watch Your Breathing

Keep your breathing regular throughout your routine. You shouldn't end a training session gasping for breath.

If you are asthmatic, don't forget to take an inhaler with you.

BALANCED LIVING: HOW TO INCORPORATE THIS EXERCISE INTO DAILY LIFE

We already know that we can do this exercise in a myriad of places. The only thing stopping us is perhaps being too shy to "make a spectacle of ourselves." You are doing this for your health and fitness, and you shouldn't worry about what outsiders think or say.

But let's have a chat about where else you can use walking on the spot:

- If you are going for a walk outside, you can include some walking-on-the-spot exercises along the way. If you know the route you will be using, select a few spots to stop and do some walking on the spot. If you don't really know your route, you can stop every 10 minutes and walk on the spot.

Walking on the spot exercises the feet, legs, and hips a little bit more than casual walking.

- Household chores can get very boring, so break it up and do some walking on the spot. For example, when you are ironing, stop and do a minute of walking on the spot after every three items. Washing dishes can also be broken up by doing some walking on the spot. When you are vacuuming the house, do some walking on the spot once you finish a room. I'm sure that now that I have given you some ideas to spark up your household chores, you can find more instances of your own.
- Bending down and gardening may strain your back, so sprinkle some walking on the spot now and then. It will help your back recover and reduce the stress on your body.
- Commercial breaks while watching TV are the perfect place to stretch yourself out by walking on the spot.
- If you are using podcasts to keep your mind active, walk on the spot so that you can exercise your mind and body together.
- Some of you may still have a job. Take frequent breaks to walk on the spot. It will revitalize your brain and stretch out your body.
- When you are standing in line at the check-out counter after doing your shopping, try to get in some walks on the spot. As you pack your groceries away, pause and do some walks.
- A cup of coffee or tea will go down well after shopping. Walk on the spot while you wait for the kettle to boil.

SEGUE

Walking on the spot is an exercise that subtly exercises so many parts of your body. It doesn't seem like much, but almost your entire body is involved in it. You practice walking by rolling your feet; this makes your feet more stable and exercises your ankles as well. Both benefits will help with any balance problems you have. Your calves and thighs will also benefit from the movement.

If you improve your posture, your hips, abs, and back will benefit. Your arms will be moving together with your legs, your right foot with your left arm, and your left foot with your right arm. You should also feel this in your shoulders and your back.

This is a simple but effective exercise to add to the others in this book. You could also use a few minutes of this exercise as a warm-up or a cool-down. It is versatile and can be done almost anywhere.

Please take note of the common errors that people make when doing this exercise and try to avoid them.

The concepts explained for this exercise can be adapted when you go for actual walks. When you are out walking concentrate on rolling your feet when you take a step. Keep the length of your step comfortable for you even if you have to take two steps for somebody else's one step.

I hope you enjoy this exercise; it is one of my favorite ones.

The next chapter deals with some more exercises that you can incorporate into your training sessions.

CHAPTER 9
MORE ADVANCED EXERCISES TO LEVEL UP YOUR ROUTINE

Wow! I am so proud of you that you have come this far. I bet when you started, you didn't think this book would help you as much as it has. How is your balance? Have you been keeping a journal of your progress? If you did, turn to the very first page where you started with split squats. Read your comments and now do a split squat. How was that now that you are so much fitter?

When you have a few spare minutes go over your journal and see for yourself just how far you have come. Be proud of yourself—I'm sorry that I don't have a star or a certificate, but you deserve both.

WHERE TO NEXT?

You are now ready to take your fitness to new levels, but don't forget about your earlier exercises. You must still incorporate them into your fitness routine as they will form your foundation. So, include about two of these per training session.

Get ready to conquer new heights in balanced living when you complete the exercises in this chapter.

ADVANCED EXERCISE #1: WALL PUSH-UPS

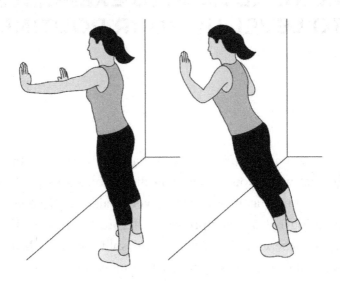

These are a bit easier than floor push-ups but have a very similar benefit. Someone once said, "Wall push-ups are regular push-ups with training wheels" (Supplements, 2022).

When you do floor push-ups you add gravity to the mix. As you extend up you are fighting gravity, so you need strong arms and a very strong core. When you do wall push-ups the fight is a bit easier as there is no problem with gravity. However, you are still engaging your arms, core, and back.

EFFECTIVE BALANCE EXERCISES FOR SENIORS   123

Why Is This Routine Essential?

A normal push-up passes through the plank position, which is difficult on your arms and shoulders. A wall push-up uses the muscles in your arms and shoulders, but there is no strain on your body. A normal pushup requires your arms and toes to take a lot.

Wall push-ups focus on the upper body, and this exercise benefits most of its muscles.

Wall push-ups help stabilize you, so your sense of balance will become better over time.

The main muscles that are engaged during this exercise are:

- chest muscles
- deltoids
- triceps
- core—these are a group of muscles extending from your front, through the sides to the back. People often think only of a six-pack when they hear the word abs.
- back muscles
- quads
- glues
- leg muscles.

If you incorporate this into your daily routine, you will soon notice a change in the definition of your muscles and strength. Your stability will also improve.

So, what can you realistically expect?

After one week:

- You will be aware of a strengthening of the stability in your upper body.
- Opening bottles may become easier as your muscles start to get stronger. You will mainly feel it in your shoulders and arms—I had very weak wrists, and surprisingly, I have felt a bit more strength there.
- Your posture will improve as long as you try to keep your body straight during the exercise.

After one month:

- The exercise will be a bit easier to achieve as your upper body gets stronger.
- You will start to receive compliments on your muscle definition.
- Your posture will improve even more.

After three months:

- You will find an improvement in your endurance.
- Your muscle definition will be obvious.
- You will experience full-body fitness.

Goals

The following is a suggestion of what you can expect when doing this exercise.

Men (50-59): Between 10 and 12 pushups

Men (60+): Between 8 and 10 pushups

Women (50-59): Between 7 and 10 pushups

Women (60+): Between 5 and 11 pushups

The Exercise

Equipment: A wall, loose clothing, and good shoes.

Remarks: Make sure that you stand the correct distance from the wall. If you are too close, it could affect your back. It could also cause injury if you are too far from the wall. Your back will be arched, and you may fall.

Instructions:

1. Face the wall. To get the correct distance stretch out your arms. Your fingertips need to be a couple of inches away from the wall. Once you have found the ideal distance, stand with your feet shoulder-width apart.
2. Lean forward to put the palms of your hands on the wall. Your hands should be shoulder-width apart and your arms straight. Your body should be inclining at about 45°.
3. Inhale as you bend your elbows as much as is comfortable. Try to get your nose as close to the wall without touching it. Keep your arms close to your body.
4. Your body should be in a straight line from your heels up to your head. Pause for a couple of seconds.
5. Exhale as you push yourself away from the wall. Push with intent until you are back to the starting position. Do not do it too quickly.

Refer to the goals section for your number of reps. Don't worry if you can't make it at first, each time you do the exercise you will get closer to your goal.

Variations

Some variations on the exercise above.

- **Intermediate:** This is very similar to the beginner version except for the foot position. To start, position your feet with the left foot a bit closer to the wall so that your feet are not next to one another. After doing half of the push-ups, take your left foot back and bring your right foot forward. This is called a split stance.
- **Advanced:** Again, this is very similar to the first one, but try to get your forearms flat against the wall.
- **Expert:** Try the single stance variation. Lift one leg while doing the push-up. Do half the number, then swap legs. It doesn't matter how high you lift your leg; you can even rest your big toe on the floor to start. As you get better you can lift your leg higher.

If you have managed to do the set number of repetitions and are beginning to get bored with the exercise, you can notch it up a bit by doing Inclined Push-ups.

1. Use a table or the kitchen counter and place your hands on the flat surface.
2. To get the right foot position, put your hands on the surface and step away until your body is straight on that incline.
3. To do the push up get on your toes and bend your arms until you are close to your chosen surface.

Benefits

Wall push-ups are easier than floor push-ups. It will just take you a bit longer to achieve your goals, but it is better for your shoulders and arms.

This exercise engages many of your muscles. It builds upper body strength but is also good for the lower body. In other words, it is almost a full-body exercise.

The stabilizer muscles in your midsection, back, and abs get a good workout, which will decrease the number of falls you may have.

Best Practices

To get the most out of your wall push-ups follow the suggestions below.

- Do the exercise slowly with control. If you do it too quickly you may lose your balance. You get more out of the exercise if you concentrate on the movement.
- Make sure not to compromise your posture. You should be simulating the plank position, which means that your entire body is involved with each movement.
- Avoid rounding your shoulders.
- Avoid arching your back. Don't collapse it keep it straight so that your body is in line all the time.
- Keep your hips in line with your back. Don't let them sag.
- Keep your head in line. Do not jut your chin forward.
- Keep your repetitions slow and steady.

Balanced Living: How to Incorporate This Exercise into Daily Life

We have already discussed many places where you can introduce exercise into your daily life. Here are some other ideas:

- When you wake up in the morning, hop out of bed and do two or three wall push-ups. A great way to get the blood coursing through your veins.
- A couple of wall push-ups are a great energy booster when the afternoon dip in energy occurs.
- As you stand waiting for the kettle to boil or for your copies to finish, throw in a couple of wall push-ups.

ADVANCED EXERCISE #2: REAR LEG LIFTS

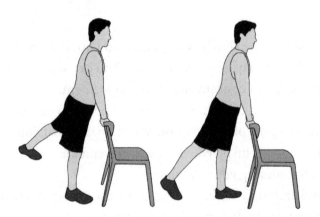

Rear Leg Lifts

Why Is This Routine Essential?

As with all the other exercises in this book, this exercise helps strengthen a variety of muscles. Even though you are lifting your leg, you exercise your abdominal muscles as well since they are needed to control the movement.

Benefits

If you incorporate this exercise into your daily exercise program, your hips, legs, and thighs will benefit. Leg raises help to stabilize you, and as you lift your leg, you will feel it in your abs as well.

After one week:

- You will find that your balance is better.

After one month:

- Your legs will be stronger, which will help your balance. You will have greater flexibility in your hips, and your posture will improve as well.

After three months:

- There will be a marked improvement in your balance as your muscles get stronger. Stronger muscles mean that you will be able to walk longer. It will increase your pain threshold.

Step-by-Step Guide to Doing Rear Leg Lifts

Equipment: Your chair.

Instructions:

1. Stand behind the chair.
2. Inhale and lift your right leg straight back as high as is comfortable. Keep your knees straight.
3. Hold—to begin with, hold the pose for one second. You can increase this as you get better at it.
4. Slowly bring your leg back down as you exhale.
5. Repeat 15 times.
6. Then repeat with your left leg.

Best Practices

The chair must be stable.

While you do the exercise, make sure that you do not compromise your posture. It is so easy to bend forward as you lift your leg. Beware of this. If you try to lift the leg too much, it might strain your back.

Balanced Living: How to Incorporate This Exercise into Daily Life

When you are taking your dog for a walk or just going for a stroll, stop at a few of the park benches and do a couple of leg lifts.

When you walk upstairs, you can hold onto the handrail and extend your leg straight back on each step. It's not quite the same, but it does feel pretty good.

ADVANCED EXERCISE #3: GET UPS

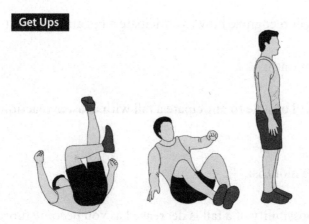

Get Ups

Why Is This Routine Essential?

This exercise combines the concepts from a few of the earlier exercises but takes it a bit further. Just a word of warning: It entails kneeling on the floor, which might be problematic for some. However, this exercise will help train you to get up after a fall. You should be toned enough by now, but just make sure you can get up from a semi-kneeling position. The exercise is complicated but very good for almost all the muscle groups.

The more you practice this, the stronger your thighs, abs, and hips will be.

This is probably the most important exercise that you need to perfect. A fall can happen at any time and anywhere. You could be with a friend or alone. You cannot just spend the rest of your days languishing on the floor; you need to get up. This exercise puts you on the floor and then helps you get back up.

After one week:

- You will recognize how to anticipate a fall and rectify it.

After one month:

- You will be able to anticipate a fall with a faster reaction time.

After three months:

- The possibility of a fall is decreased as you become more aware of your feelings.

Step-by-Step Guide to Do Get-Ups

Equipment: You may like to have a counter or your chair close by in case you need it.

Instructions:

1. By now, you will know which leg is your dominant one. Put all your weight onto that leg and move the other leg backward as far as you feel comfortable. Put your hands on the thigh of the front leg.

2. Bend your back leg until it is kneeling on the floor. Do this slowly and with control. Use your abs to stabilize the position. You can use the chair to help you stabilize.

3. Keep one hand on your thigh and bring the other hand to the floor next to the front foot. Your abs will support your spine.

4. Bring your front leg back so that you are kneeling on all fours. Your hands on the floor should be under your shoulders and your knees should be under your hips. Engage your core to help stabilize yourself.

5. Twist your body to whichever side is easiest. Let your hip touch the floor. If you wish you can adjust your knees so that you are sitting on the floor.

6. So now you are on the floor, and you need to get up. This procedure is the reverse of what you did to get on the floor.

- Get onto all fours again.
- Bring your dominant leg forward with a bent knee.
- Place both hands on the thigh of your dominant leg. You can use the toes of your back leg to help you by curling them under.
- Push your hands down and use your thigh and your upper body to get back to a standing position.

7. Bring your feet together in preparation for repeating the exercise.

Remember you have the chair to help you if you get stuck. This is very important exercise as there is nothing worse than getting stuck on the floor if you fall. So, to summarize it quickly: Get into a kneeling position and move to sit on the floor. Get back to the kneeling position and then stand up. Seems simple now, doesn't it?

It will get easier as you practice it, and it will take away your fear of falling.

How to Incorporate This Exercise into Daily Life

I used to love sitting or lying on the floor. I would watch TV from the floor or lie on my stomach, reading my favorite book of the moment. I would sit cross-legged on the floor to do my art. I would sort out my papers on the floor. There was so much space to do all of these tasks, and then, gradually, it began to get a bit harder. Then, harder still, until one day, I was stuck on the floor. I had to crawl to a chair so that I had something to help me get up. Alas, my floor days are over. But now that I have learned this exercise, I may be back on the floor again.

There is one obvious way that you can use this exercise and that is just fall! But I won't wish that on you. So, let's examine some other ways that you can use this around and about.

- When gardening, it is pleasant to sit on the grass and weed nearby. Use the first part of the exercise to get down on the grass. Do what you have to do down there, and then use the second part of the exercise to get back up.
- Think about the last time that you went to the beach. Were you sitting on a deck chair while everyone else was enjoying the fun of being on the sand and building sandcastles while you sat there watching them? Well, next time you go to the beach, you can join them in the sand.
- Now, just for fun: Get your favorite book and lie down on the floor to read it. Then, you have to get back up at some point.
- The next time you have papers to sort, get down on the floor and get back up after you have finished.
- Get down to your pet's level and roll around on the floor with them.

- There is a funny saying for seniors: If you have to get down on the floor, crawl around on the floor and do everything that you need to do while on the floor, such as picking up papers. While you are down there, you might as well do everything that has to be done down there.

This was a bonus chapter. The other eight chapters deal with one exercise per chapter. Chapter 9 has given you three extra exercises and some breathing exercises. All of them are quite important. The exercises here are quite useful in helping your stability and your posture.

Whole books have been written on wall exercises, and the most important one is the first one in this chapter. Wall push-ups are much easier than floor Push-ups yet they have almost the same benefits. Push-ups—wall or otherwise—exercise almost all your muscles.

Rear leg lifts help the muscles around your midriff as long as you do not compromise your posture. It is very easy to tilt forward as you lift your leg back, but you won't get much benefit from that. If you make sure that your chin is always parallel to the ground, it will be hard to compromise your posture. At first, you won't get your leg very high, but the more you do the exercise, the higher you will get your leg.

The last exercise is a very important one as it teaches your body how to react if you fall. In the exercise, you are purposely getting down on the floor. The technique of getting down on the floor is not as important as the technique of getting up. You can use it when you get on the floor on purpose like when you do some gardening. If you fall, do some gardening, or lie down on the beach you are going to need to get up. You can adapt the technique described here in any situation.

Make a Difference!

In the space of just a few minutes, you could make a massive difference to someone else's quality of life.

Simply by sharing your honest opinion of this book and a little about your own experience, you'll help other people who are looking for guidance on improving their balance find exactly the advice they need to help them.

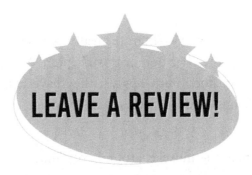

Thank you so much for your support. It might not feel like much, but it could make a huge difference to someone else's life.

Scan the QR code to leave a review:

CONCLUSION

Congratulations on making it to the end of this book. I sincerely hope that you are enjoying your exercise time and that your condition has improved.

POSSIBLE IMPROVEMENTS

Although the exercises that I have selected are primarily for balance, they also have some other takeaways:

- Any exercise you do at any stage of life will help you get fit. However, it is more important to get fit when you are a senior. Fitness can be equated to a superb quality of life.
- You will find that you are less dependent on others. As you age, it is important that you retain as much independence as possible. You don't want to be a drain on your family.
- You may have been reticent to get out and about because you had no confidence in yourself. When you see how fit you are, going out for any reason will not bother you. You might not enjoy shopping trips, but you will no longer

dread them. Going out with friends or family will be pleasurable once your fear of losing your balance has gone.

- You will be less tired during the day since your stamina has improved.

This book has hopefully answered many of your concerns and has given you the following takeaways.

Watch Your Step

I don't mean that you could get into trouble! You must literally watch your step, where you put your feet, for trip hazards, and take care when you walk on gravel or an uneven pathway. If you misstep, you could end up falling or twisting your ankle.

Stand Strong

By now, you will be able to stand without wobbling. Your legs, ankles, and feet have increased strength, which will allow you to stand for much longer periods. Your stance will also be stronger.

Make it Fun

When you exercise, it is easy to become bored. Swapping the exercises around will fight this tendency. Make your exercise sessions fun so that you will be eager to start every day.

Keep a Log

You might not think that this is necessary, but keeping a log has a few advantages.

- It clarifies any problems you may have in understanding the instructions of the exercises.
- It highlights your improvements when you compare today's session with the first session. If you compare today's session with yesterday's session, you may pick up problems that you have overcome.
- You can use it to bolster your feelings of success. It can be used whenever you are feeling down because a session went badly or when you feel you are not achieving anything. Looking back will make you realize that you have actually accomplished great things since you first started.
- It also adds discipline to your exercise session. When you are disciplined to write a session up, you can be sure that you maintain discipline throughout your session.

You could keep a physical log in a book, or you can do a virtual log using a word processor.

Reward Yourself

It is very important to reward yourself when you have had a good session, or you have achieved a goal. You could establish goals in your journal, and when you have achieved them, you can reward yourself. Remember that rewards should not be in the form of food, snacks, or sweets. It is something that is prevalent in all cultures, for example:

- It's your birthday so we must have a feast.
- You passed your exam let's go out to dinner.
- You won your race so here's a box of chocolates.

Rather reward yourself with things that you wouldn't necessarily buy yourself like:

- a spa treatment
- the latest best-seller
- a magazine subscription
- a new outfit
- a new pair of shoes
- a day off
- a movie or a theatrical performance

Think what you would like as a reward, and under which conditions you will reward yourself and jot it down in your journal.

Don't let people define you by your age. You are so much more than that. Rather, encourage them to define you by your actions and successes. You can define yourself by reaching personal goals. Your improved balance can define you.

SUMMARY OF THE EXERCISES

For convenience. I am including a summary of the exercises just in case you want to refer to them again and can't remember where to find them. The table also includes the main benefits, so if you want to find which exercise, for example, strengthens your ankles, you can pick that up in the benefits column.

Remember, as your core strengthens, your posture will improve, and your lower body will strengthen.

Chapter	Exercise	Benefits
Chapter 2	Split Squats	Joint and muscle development
Chapter 3	Chair Raises	Improved balance and core development
Chapter 4	Single Leg Stance	Enhanced stability and increased strength in the lower body
Chapter 5	Shin Exercises	Strengthens the lower body, particularly the ankles
Chapter 6	Calf Raises	Improved balance and enhanced strength of the ankles and calves
Chapter 7	Heel to Toe Walk	Enhanced balance as the ankles are made stronger
Chapter 8	Marching in Place	Improves blood circulation and strengthens the lower body which in turn will increase stability
Chapter 9 (1)	Wall Push-ups	Gives you a complete body workout and helps your posture and balance
Chapter 9 (2)	Rear Leg Lifts	Improves your balance and posture as well as your endurance and mobility
Chapter 9 (3)	Get Ups	This exercise teaches you how to get up if you happen to fall. If you feel dizzy and you think you may fall, you can use the movements to lessen your impact with the floor, and when you have stabilized yourself, you can use the second part of this exercise to get back up.

ACHIEVEMENTS

You have followed every exercise in this book. Sometimes it has been tough, and sometimes it has been easy, but you have persevered. You have seen the difference that your dedication to a better body and better balance has given you. Your body has been reshaped, and you can now walk with confidence without worrying about falling. And if you do trip and fall, the get-ups exercise will help lessen the impact and help you get up again.

Now that you have made a positive impact on your body keep it up. If you carry on with the exercises given here, your senior years will truly be your golden years. Your friends and others who are your age or maybe even younger than you will be envious of your agility and will want to know your secret.

When your friends see the changes in you, encourage them to make a positive move to better their lives. Share the fact that, for you, these exercises have become a way of life and that you have learned how to incorporate the techniques into your day. Explain that you try to set aside half an hour a day to devote to your well-being, and if you don't have the time on a particular day, you know how to build the exercises into your life as you go about the chores of that day. The exercises have redefined you as you represent the new, flexible you to them.

WRAP UP

If you feel you have gained a whole new perspective on your life with this book, you need to share the information. Just think, you could help someone who is battling the same battles you were before you found this book.

Could you leave a review explaining how this book changed your life? The review may reach someone desperate to make changes that will help their balance, posture, stability, and well-being.

REFERENCES

Ade, V., Schalkwijk, D., Psarakis, M., Laporte, M. D., Faras, T. J., Sandoval, R., Najjar, F., & Stubbs, P. W. (2018). Between session reliability of heel-to-toe progression measurements in the stance phase of gait. *PLOS ONE, 13*(7), e0200436. https://doi.org/10.1371/journal.pone.0200436

American Heart Association. (2014). *Balance Exercise.* Heart.org. https://www.heart.org/en/healthy-living/fitness/fitness-basics/balance-exercise

American Sports and Fitness Association. (2022). *Golden Age Fitness: Exercise Tips for Older Adults.* ASFA. https://www.americansportandfitness.com/blogs/fitness-blog/golden-age-fitness-exercise-tips-for-older-adults

Anderson, A. R. (2016, May 31). *The Importance Of Having Balance In Our Lives.* Forbes. https://www.forbes.com/sites/amyanderson/2016/05/31/the-importance-of-having-balance-in-our-lives/?sh=5deb82a2a93e

Araujo, C. G., de Souza e Silva, C. G., Laukkanen, J. A., Fiatarone Singh, M., Kunutsor, S., Myers, J., Franca, J. F., & Castro, C. L. (2022). Successful 10-second one-legged stance performance predicts survival in middle-aged and older individuals. *British Journal of Sports Medicine*, bjsports-2021-105360. https://doi.org/10.1136/bjsports-2021-105360

armchairpugilist. (2016, August 26). *Older people who were very physically active earlier in life, how has that changed?* Reddit. https://www.reddit.com/r/AskOldPeople/comments/4znbqm/older_people_who_were_very_physically_active/?rdt=62851

ASFA. (2022b). *The Importance of Flexibility and Function in Daily Life.* https://www.americansportandfitness.com/blogs/fitness-blog/the-importance-of-flexibility-and-function-in-daily-life

Better Health. (2021). *Physical activity - how to get active when you are busy.* https://www.betterhealth.vic.gov.au/health/HealthyLiving/Physical-activity-how-to-get-active-when-you-are-busy

Better Health Channel. (2015). *Ageing - muscles bones and joints.* https://www.betterhealth.vic.gov.au/health/conditionsandtreatments/ageing-muscles-bones-and-joints

Bhardwaj, N. (2020, February 26). *These 5 benefits of calf raises will make you want to do the exercise ASAP.* Healthshots. https://www.healthshots.com/fitness/muscle-gain/5-benefits-of-calf-raises/

Boston Children's Hospital. (2023). *Broken Tibia-Fibula (Shinbone/Calf Bone).*

https://www.childrenshospital.org/conditions/broken-tibia-fibula-shin bonecalf-bone

Bumgardner, W. (2021, October 19). *10 Walking Mistakes to Avoid*. Verywell Fit. https://www.verywellfit.com/walking-mistakes-to-avoid-3435576

CaroMont Health. (2021, September 26). *Seven Easy Ways to Include Exercise in Your Daily Routine*. https://caromonthealth.org/news/seven-easy-ways-to-include-exercise-in-your-daily-routine/

CDC. (2017). *30-Second Chair Stand*. Centers for Disease Control and Prevention. https://www.cdc.gov/steadi/pdf/STEADI-Assessment-30Sec-508.pdf

CDC. (2020a, January 8). *Making Physical Activity a Part of an Older Adult's Life*. Centers for Disease Control and Prevention. https://www.cdc.gov/physicalactivity/basics/adding-pa/activities-olderadults.htm

CDC. (2020b, December 16). *Keep on Your Feet*. Centers for Disease Control and Prevention. https://www.cdc.gov/injury/features/older-adult-falls/index.html

CDC. (2021, August 6). *Facts about falls*. Centers for Disease Control and Prevention. https://www.cdc.gov/falls/facts.html

CDC. (2023). *Stay independent*. Centers for Disease Control and Prevention. https://www.cdc.gov/steadi/pdf/STEADI-Brochure-StayIndependent-508.pdf

CDC. (2019). *How much physical activity do older adults need?* Centers for Disease Control and Prevention. https://www.cdc.gov/physicalactivity/basics/older_adults/index.htm

CDC. (2021, November 1). Centers for Disease Control and Prevention. *Benefits of Physical Activity*. CDC.https://www.cdc.gov/physicalactivity/basics/pa-health/index.htm

Chubb, P. (2023). *5 Reasons Why You Should Do Split Squats*. Mindful Mover. https://mindfulmover.com/5-reasons-why-you-should-do-split-squats/

Clarity Clinic. (2019, June 10). *In-Person & Online Therapy and Psychiatric Services*. https://www.claritychi.com/blog/balancing-aspects-of-life

Clear, J. (2018, July 13). *How Long Does It Actually Take to Form a New Habit? (Backed by Science)*. James Clear. https://jamesclear.com/new-habit

Cronkleton, E. (2019, April 9). *10 Breathing Techniques*. Healthline. https://www.healthline.com/health/breathing-exercise

Cronkleton, E. (2020, July 28). *Never Skip a Leg Day: Benefits, Cautions, and More*. Healthline. https://www.healthline.com/health/exercise-fitness/never-skip-leg-day

Dale, M. (2022). *March: Ten Variations for Marching*. MusiKinesis. https://www.musikinesis.com/ideas-to-try/two-movement-ideas-for-march/

Deshmukh, N. S., & Phansopkar, P. (2022). *Medial Tibial Stress Syndrome: A Review Article*. Cureus, *14(7)*. https://doi.org/10.7759/cureus.26641

Emilio, E. J. M.-L., Hita-Contreras, F., Jiménez-Lara, P. M., Latorre-Román, P., &

Martínez-Amat, A. (2014). The association of flexibility, balance, and lumbar strength with balance ability: risk of falls in older adults. *Journal of Sports Science & Medicine, 13*(2), 349–357. https://www.ncbi.nlm.nih.gov/pmc/arti cles/PMC3990889/

Evers, C. (2022, May 1). *How Standing Calf Raises Help You Stay Strong & Stable.* Verywell Fit. https://www.verywellfit.com/how-to-do-calf-raises-4801090

Farnsworth, L. (2021, June 23). *The Connection between Strength, Flexibility, and Balance.* Observing Leslie. https://observingleslie.com/magazine/the-connec tion-between-strength-flexibility-and-balance

Fitness Together. (2023). *The Low-Impact Benefits of a March-in-Place Workout.* https://fitnesstogether.com/ellicottcity/blog/the-low-impact-benefits-of-a-march-in-place-workout

Fletcher, J. (2019, February 12). *4-7-8 breathing: How it works, benefits, and uses.* Medical News Today. https://www.medicalnewstoday.com/articles/324417

Health Essentials. (2018, October 24). *How You Can Fix a Dowager's Hump + Prevention Tips.* Cleveland Clinic. https://health.clevelandclinic.org/how-you-can-fix-a-dowagers-hump-prevention-tips/

Health System University of Michigan. (2016). *Balance Exercises Static Standing - Single Leg Stance.* https://www.med.umich.edu/1libr/PMR/BalanceExercises/StaticStanding_SingleLeg.pdf

Healthwise Staff. (2022, November 9). *Shin Splints (Shin Pain): Exercises.* My Health Alberta. https://myhealth.alberta.ca/Health/aftercareinformation/pages/condi tions.aspx?hwid=bo1640

Healthwise Staff. (2023, March 1). *Marching-in-Place Exercise to Improve Balance.* My Health Alberta. https://myhealth.alberta.ca/Health/pages/conditions.aspx?hwid=zm2304

Inverarity, L. (2021, July 5). *Improve Your Balance With the Single Leg Stance Exercise.* Verywell Fit. https://www.verywellfit.com/single-leg-stance-exercise-for-better-balance-2696233

Kinship Pointe. (2021, December 9). *Why Flexibility Is Important for Seniors.* https://kinshippointe.com/why-flexibility-is-important-for-seniors/

LetsPlayKvetch. (2018, July 17). *What's been the most difficult physical part about getting older?* Reddit. https://www.reddit.com/r/RedditForGrownups/comments/8zjs8z/whats_been_the_most_difficult_physical_part_about/

Liberty Homecare and Hospice. (2021, October 6). *At-Home Exercises for Older Adults.* https://libertyhomecare.com/at-home-exercises-for-older-adults/

Lien, P. (2021, May 11). *Coronavirus Recovery: Breathing Exercises.* Hopkins Medicine. https://www.hopkinsmedicine.org/health/conditions-and-diseases/coronavirus/coronavirus-recovery-breathing-exercises

Lutsiv, N. (2022, December 12). *Is Walking In Place A Good Exercise?* BetterMe Blog.

https://betterme.world/articles/is-walking-in-place-good-exercise/

Madison. (2021, January 18). *How To Manage Balance Problems In Seniors.* Meetcaregivers.com. https://meetcaregivers.com/balance-problems-in-seniors/

Marcori, A. J., Monteiro, P. H. M., Oliveira, J. A., Doumas, M., & Teixeira, L. A. (2022). Single Leg Balance Training: A Systematic Review. *Perceptual and Motor Skills, 129*(2), 232–252. https://doi.org/10.1177/00315125211070104

Maresova, P., Javanmardi, E., Barakovic, S., Barakovic Husic, J., Tomsone, S., Krejcar, O., & Kuca, K. (2019). Consequences of chronic diseases and other limitations associated with old age – a scoping review. *BMC Public Health, 19*(1). https://doi.org/10.1186/s12889-019-7762-5

Martin, M. (2011, February 7). *Single Leg Balance Exercise with Movement.* MelioGuide. https://melioguide.com/balance-exercises-for-seniors/single-leg-balance-exercises-for-older-adults/

MoreLifeHealth. (2022). *Seated Calf Raise Exercises.* https://morelifehealth.com/seated-calf-raises

Mosley, M. (2023). *Just One Thing with Michael Mosley - Why you should stand on one leg.* BBC. https://www.bbc.co.uk/programmes/articles/35QytBYmkXJ4JnDYl9zYngb/why-you-should-stand-on-one-leg

Move It or Lose It. (2017, December 4). *Can you...? Get up from the floor easily.* https://www.moveitorloseit.co.uk/can-get-floor-easily/

Naidoo, S. (n.d.). *Calf Exercises For Seniors And The Elderly.* Eldergym. https://eldergym.com/calf-exercises/

National Heart, Lung, and Blood Institute. (2022, March 24). *Physical Activity and Your Heart - Benefits.* https://www.nhlbi.nih.gov/health/heart/physical-activity/benefits

National Institute on Aging. (2020, April 2). *Four Types of Exercise Can Improve Your Health and Physical Ability.* https://www.nia.nih.gov/health/four-types-exercise-can-improve-your-health-and-physical-ability

National Institute on Aging. (2022, September 12). *Older Adults and Balance Problems.* https://www.nia.nih.gov/health/older-adults-and-balance-problems

National Institute on Aging. (2023, January 25). *Talking With Your Older Patients.* https://www.nia.nih.gov/health/health-care-professionals-information/talking-your-older-patients

Nelson, C. (2020, January 9). *The Ultimate Muscle Groups Guide & How To Best Train Them.* Levels. https://levelsprotein.com/blogs/guides/the-ultimate-muscle-groups-guide

NHS. (2017, October 17). *Balance exercises.* https://www.nhs.uk/live-well/exercise/strength-and-flexibility-exercises/balance-exercises/

Ortiz, D. (2020, August 5). *7 Causes of Balance Issues in the Golden Years.* Home Care

Assistance of Jefferson County. https://www.homecareassistancejeffersonco. com/what-can-be-causing-my-elderly-parents-balance-difficulties/

Physiopedia. (2012). *Balance.* https://www.physio-pedia.com/Balance

Physiopedia. (2019). *30 Seconds Sit to Stand Test.* https://www.physio-pedia.com/ 30_Seconds_Sit_To_Stand_Test

Piedmont Orthopedics. (2023). *5 Easy Stretches to Prevent Shin Splints.* OrthoAtlanta. https://www.orthoatlanta.com/media/5-easy-stretches-to-prevent-shin-splints

Possamai Menezes, L., Stamm, B., Tambara Leite, M., Hildebrandt, L. M., & Kirchner, R. M. (2016). Cair faz parte da vida: Fatores de risco para quedas em idosos Falling is a part of life: Falls risk factors to the elderly. *Revista de Pesquisa Cuidado é Fundamental Online, 8*(4), 5080–5086. https://doi.org/10.9789/2175-5361.2016.v8i4.5080-5086

Rai, A. (2023, January 12). Why Maintaining Mental Balance is the Need of the Hour. *The Times of India.* https://timesofindia.indiatimes.com/readersblog/ arihantsweekly/why-maintaining-mental-balance-is-the-need-of-the-hour-49118/

Rebecca Buffum Taylor. (2011, June 29). *Calf-Strengthening Exercises.* WebMD; WebMD. https://www.webmd.com/fitness-exercise/strengthening-calf-muscles

Rehab 2 Perform. (2021, February 18). *4 Hidden Benefits of Single-Leg Training.* https://rehab2perform.com/news/benefits-single-leg-training/

Ryan, S. (2013, May 20). *30 Second Sit to Stand Test.* https://www.sralab.org/rehabili tation-measures/30-second-sit-stand-test

senior_admin00. (2023, April 30). *Walking Tall: The Importance of Heel-to-Toe Walks for Senior Fall Prevention.* Senior Exercises. https://seniorexercises.fit/fitness/ walking-tall-the-importance-of-heel-to-toe-walks-for-senior-fall-prevention/

Sitthiracha, P., Eungpinichpong, W., & Chatchawan, U. (2021). Effect of Progressive Step Marching Exercise on Balance Ability in the Elderly: A Cluster Randomized Clinical Trial. *International Journal of Environmental Research and Public Health, 18*(6), 3146. https://doi.org/10.3390/ijerph18063146

Spark People. (n.d.). *How to Walk with Proper Form and Technique for Fitness.* https:// www.maine.gov/mdot/challengeme/topics/docs/2019/may/How-to-Walk-with-Proper-Form-and-Technique-for-Fitness.pdf

SportsInjuryClinic. (2020, May 2). *Shin Splints Exercises.* https://www.sportsin juryclinic.net/sport-injuries/lower-leg/shin-pain/shin-splints-exercises

Spotebi. (2015, February 26). *March In Place.* https://www.spotebi.com/exercise-guide/march-in-place/

Stathokostas, L., Little, R. M. D., Vandervoort, A. A., & Paterson, D. H. (2012). Flexibility Training and Functional Ability in Older Adults: A Systematic

Review. *Journal of Aging Research, 2012,* 1–30. https://doi.org/10.1155/2012/306818

Stefanacci, R. G., & Wilkinson, J. R. (2023, November). *Falls in Older Adults.* MSD Manual Professional Edition. https://www.msdmanuals.com/professional/geriatrics/falls-in-older-adults/falls-in-older-adults?autoredirectid=22738

Sturm-Ornezeder, T. (2022, April 27). *Walking Technique: Heel Strike, Toe Strike, and Posture.* Adidas Runtastic Blog. https://www.runtastic.com/blog/en/walking-technique/

Steel Supplements. (2022, October 24). *How to Do Wall Push Ups (Form & Benefits).* https://steelsupplements.com/blogs/steel-blog/how-to-do-wall-push-ups-form-benefits

Suzi. (2021, March 15). *You Have to Learn to Walk Before You Can Run.* Confessions of a Fitness Instructor. https://confessionsofafitnessinstructor.com/2021/03/walk-before-run/

Taylor, M. (2022, July 3). *Over 60? Walk This Way Every Day.* Livestrong.com. https://www.livestrong.com/article/13771073-heel-toe-walking/

Thiamwong, L., & Suwanno, J. (2014). Effects of Simple Balance Training on Balance Performance and Fear of Falling in Rural Older Adults. *International Journal of Gerontology, 8*(3), 143–146. https://doi.org/10.1016/j.ijge.2013.08.011

Tom. (2021, October 12). *Tibialis Raises: A simple yet powerful knee strengthening exercise.* Energy for Life Fitness. https://www.energyforlifefitness.com/protect-your-knees-with-tibialis-riases/

Topend Sports. (2019). *2 Minute Step in Place Test.* https://www.topendsports.com/testing/tests/step-in-place-2min.htm

University of Michigan. (2016). *Physical Medicine and Rehabilitation Walking Exercises G-13: Heel to Toe Walk Forward.* https://www.med.umich.edu/1libr/PMR/BalanceExercises/Gait_TandemForward.pdf

Veda. (2023). *Balance & Aging.* Vestibular Disorders Association. https://vestibular.org/article/coping-support/living-with-a-vestibular-disorder/age-related-dizziness-and-imbalance/balance-aging/

Vincent, Sarah. *50 Quotes About Aging That Make You Feel Good About Getting Older.* Reader's Digest. Last modified January 31, 2024. https://www.rd.com/article/quotes-about-aging/

Waehner, P. (2019, August 30). *How to Safely Get up and Down From the Floor.* Verywell Fit. https://www.verywellfit.com/how-to-safely-get-up-and-down-from-the-floor-1230957

Waida, M. (2020, October 28). *Top Tips for Incorporating Exercise Into Daily Life | Wrike.* Blog Wrike. https://www.wrike.com/blog/how-to-fit-exercise-into-a-busy-schedule/

WebMD. (2022a, July 21). *How to Do Split Squats.* https://www.webmd.com/ fitness-exercise/how-to-do-split-squats

WebMD. (2022b, August 17). *What's Normal Aging and What Can You Do About It?* https://www.webmd.com/healthy-aging/normal-aging

wikiHow (30 Jan 2021). *How to Exercise Your Shin Muscles.* [Video]. YouTube. https://www.youtube.com/watch?v=yqVeC3n1CbQ

World Health Organization. (2021). *Falls.* https://www.who.int/news-room/fact-sheets/detail/falls

World Health Organization. (2023, February 21). *Stress.* https://www.who.int/ news-room/questions-and-answers/item/stress

Zorzan, N. (2022, October 31). *Best chair exercises for seniors: Safe and easy workouts.* Medical News Today. https://www.medicalnewstoday.com/articles/chair-exer cises-for-seniors#neck-rotations

Made in the USA
Middletown, DE
02 January 2025

68670572R00086